# Food Science and Nutrition:
# An Integrated Approach

# Food Science and Nutrition: An Integrated Approach

Reese Burnett

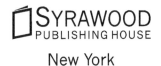

SYRAWOOD
PUBLISHING HOUSE

New York

Published by Syrawood Publishing House,
750 Third Avenue, 9th Floor,
New York, NY 10017, USA
www.syrawoodpublishinghouse.com

**Food Science and Nutrition: An Integrated Approach**
Reese Burnett

International Standard Book Number: 978-1-64740-150-4 (Hardback)

This book contains information obtained from authentic and highly regarded sources. All chapters are published with permission under the Creative Commons Attribution Share Alike License or equivalent. A wide variety of references are listed. Permissions and sources are indicated; for detailed attributions, please refer to the permissions page. Reasonable efforts have been made to publish reliable data and information, but the authors, editors and publisher cannot assume any responsibility for the validity of all materials or the consequences of their use.

**Trademark Notice:** Registered trademark of products or corporate names are used only for explanation and identification without intent to infringe.

**Cataloging-in-Publication Data**

Food science and nutrition : an integrated approach / Reese Burnett.
    p. cm.
Includes bibliographical references and index.
ISBN 978-1-64740-150-4
1. Food. 2. Nutrition. 3. Food--Technology. 4. Food industry and trade.
5. Diet. I. Burnett, Reese.
TX357 .F66 2022
641.3--dc23

# Table of Contents

# Preface

This book is a culmination of my many years of practice in this field. I attribute the success of this book to my support group. I would like to thank my parents who have showered me with unconditional love and support and my peers and professors for their constant guidance.

Food science deals with the study of food. It is an interdisciplinary field that encompasses engineering, biological and physical sciences. It uses all such fields to study the nature of foods, causes of deterioration, principles of food processing as well as the improvement of food in order to make it ready for consumption. Food science is also involved in the development of new food products, designing of processes that are used to produce these foods, choosing packaging materials, shelf-life studies as well as microbiological and chemical testing. It applies concepts from various fields such as chemistry, microbiology, biochemistry and physiology. This book attempts to understand the multiple aspects of food science and nutrition, and how such concepts have practical applications. It is appropriate for students seeking detailed information in this area as well as for experts. Coherent flow of topics, student-friendly language and extensive use of examples make this book an invaluable source of knowledge.

The details of chapters are provided below for a progressive learning:

Chapter – Introduction

The branch of science which deals with the study of nature of food, causes for deterioration, its processing and improvement for consumption. Nutrition refers to the process of taking up of nutrients and using them for growth, metabolism, and repair of body. This is an introductory chapter which will briefly introduce about food science and nutrition.

Chapter – Branches of Food Science

The field of food science can be branched into 4 major divisions. It includes food chemistry, food engineering, food technology and food microbiology. This chapter has been carefully written to provide an easy understanding of these branches of food science.

Chapter – Nutrients

The nutrients can be broadly classified into two categories, namely, micronutrients and macronutrients. Some of the micronutrients are vitamins and minerals while carbohydrates, proteins and fats fall under macronutrients. This chapter discusses about these different types of essential nutrients in detail.

Chapter – Common Food Additives

Food additive refers to a chemical substance which is added to food in order to enhance the taste, appearance and preserve its flavor. Anticaking agents, food coloring and glazing agents are a few examples of commonly used food additives. The diverse applications of these additives have been thoroughly discussed in this chapter.

Chapter – Food Contamination

Food contamination is the presence of harmful chemicals and microorganisms in food which can cause food-borne illnesses. Biological contamination, physical contamination, chemical contamination, etc. fall under its domain. The topics elaborated in this chapter will help in gaining a better perspective about these aspects related to food contamination.

Chapter – Food Preservation

Food preservation is defined as the prevention of the growth of microorganisms and maintain food quality. It includes some methods such as fermentation, pasteurization, salting, pickling, canning, salting, etc. This chapter closely examines these methods of food preservation to provide an extensive understanding of the subject.

**Reese Burnett**

# 1
# Introduction

The branch of science which deals with the study of nature of food, causes for deterioration, its processing and improvement for consumption. Nutrition refers to the process of taking up of nutrients and using them for growth, metabolism, and repair of body. This is an introductory chapter which will briefly introduce about food science and nutrition.

## Food Science

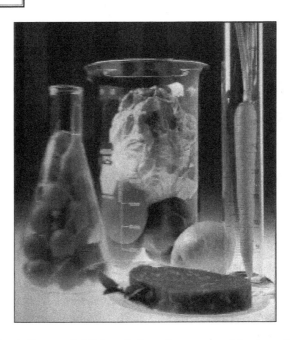

Food Science is a multi-disciplinary field involving chemistry, biochemistry, nutrition, microbiology and engineering to give one the scientific knowledge to solve real problems associated with the many facets of the food system. The basis of the discipline lies in an understanding of the chemistry of food components, such as proteins, carbohydrates, fats and water and the reactions they undergo during processing and storage. A complete understanding of processing and preservation methods is required including drying, freezing, pasteurization, canning, irradiation, extrusion, to name just a few. The ability to carry out analysis of food constituents is developed along with statistical quality control methods. The microbiology and the safety aspects of food must also be understood. Other topics covered include food additives, the physico-chemical properties of food, flavor chemistry, product development, food engineering and packaging. Food science integrates this broad-based knowledge and focuses it on food.

Food Science is still a relatively new and growing discipline, brought about mainly as a response to the social changes taking place in North America and other parts of the developed world. The food industry, which originally provided only primary products for final preparation in the home, finds itself responding to market demands for more refined, sophisticated, and convenient products. The demand for easy to prepare, convenience foods, poses major scientific and technological challenges which cannot be met without highly trained scientists capable of understanding the complex chemistry/biochemistry of food systems and knowledge of the methods to preserve them. This increased reliance of society on ready-to-eat foods has led to greater responsibility for processors in terms of quality, safety and nutrition. In order to ensure high quality and competitive products, scientific principles and new technologies are being applied to food manufacturing and the body of knowledge required has become that discipline called Food Science.

# Nutrition

Nutrition is the assimilation by living organisms of food materials that enable them to grow, maintain themselves, and reproduce.

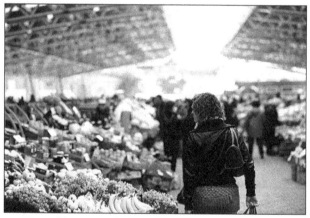
Vegetables are an important part of a balanced diet.

Food serves multiple functions in most living organisms. For example, it provides materials that are metabolized to supply the energy required for the absorption and translocation of nutrients, for the synthesis of cell materials, for movement and locomotion, for excretion of waste products, and for all other activities of the organism. Food also provides materials from which all the structural and catalytic components of the living cell can be assembled. Living organisms differ in the particular substances that they require as food, in the manner in which they synthesize food substances or obtain them from the surrounding environment, and in the functions that these substances carry out in their cells. Nevertheless, general patterns can be discerned in the nutritional process throughout the living world and in the types of nutrients that are required to sustain life.

MyPlate, a revised set of dietary guidelines introduced by the U.S. Department of Agriculture in 2011, divides the four basic food groups (fruits, grains, protein, and vegetables) into sections on a plate, with the size of each section representing the relative dietary proportions of each food group. The small blue circle shown at the upper right illustrates the inclusion and recommended proportion of dairy products in the diet.

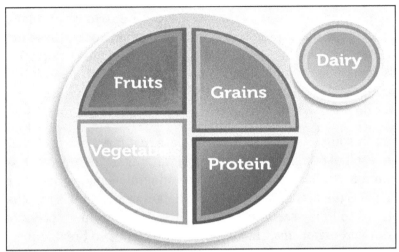

MyPlate; dietary guidelines, U.S. Department of Agriculture.

## Nutritional Patterns in the Living World

Living organisms can be categorized by the way in which the functions of food are carried out in their bodies. Thus, organisms such as green plants and some bacteria that need only inorganic compounds for growth can be called autotrophic organisms; and organisms, including all animals, fungi, and most bacteria, that require both inorganic and organic compounds for growth are called heterotrophic. Other classifications have been used to include various other nutritional patterns. In one scheme, organisms are classified according to the energy source they utilize. Phototrophic, or photosynthetic, organisms trap light energy and convert it to chemical energy, whereas chemoautotrophic, or chemosynthetic, organisms utilize inorganic or organic compounds to supply their energy requirements. If the electron-donor materials utilized to form reduced coenzymes consist of inorganic compounds, the organism is said to be lithotrophic; if organic, the organism is organotrophic.

Combinations of these patterns may also be used to describe organisms. Higher plants, for example, are photolithotrophic; i.e., they utilize light energy, with the inorganic compound water serving as the ultimate electron donor. Certain photosynthetic bacteria that cannot utilize water as the electron donor and require organic compounds for this purpose are called photoorganotrophs. Animals, according to this classification, are chemoorganotrophs; i.e., they utilize chemical compounds to supply energy and organic compounds as electron donors.

Despite wide variations in the nature of the external energy source utilized by various organisms, all organisms form from their external energy source an immediate source of energy, the chemical compound adenosine triphosphate (ATP). This energy-rich compound is common to all cells. Through the breaking of its high-energy phosphate bonds and thus by its conversion to a less energy-rich compound, adenosine diphosphate (ADP), ATP provides the energy for the chemical and mechanical work required by an organism. The energy requirements of organisms can be measured in either joules or calories.

## Nutrition in Plants

Plants, unlike animals, do not have to obtain organic materials for their nutrition, although these form the bulk of their tissues. By trapping solar energy in photosynthetic systems, they are able to synthesize nutrients from carbon dioxide ($CO_2$) and water. However, plants do require inorganic salts, which they absorb from the soil surrounding their roots; these include the elements phosphorus (in the form of phosphate), chlorine (as the chloride ion), potassium, sulfur, calcium, magnesium, iron, manganese, boron, copper, and zinc. Plants also require nitrogen, in the form of nitrate ($NO_3^-$) or ammonium ($NH_4^+$) ions. They will, in addition, take up inorganic compounds that they themselves do not need, such as iodides and cobalt and selenium salts.

The nutrients found in soil result in part from the gradual breakdown of the rocky material on Earth's surface as a result of rain and, in some areas, freezing. Primarily composed of alumina and silica, rocks also contain smaller amounts of all the mineral elements needed by plants. Another source of soil nutrients is the decomposition of dead plants and animals and their waste products. Although a spadeful of soil may seem inert to the eye—apart from an occasional earthworm—it contains millions of microorganisms, the net effect of which is to break down organic materials, releasing simpler mineral salts. Furthermore, two groups of bacteria fix atmospheric nitrogen— that is, they are able to incorporate this relatively inert element into nitrate ions. Bacteria of the genus Azobacter live freely in soil, while those of the genus Rhizobium live sheltered in the roots of leguminous plants such as peas and beans. Cyanobacteria (blue-green algae) also can fix nitrogen and are important for growing rice in the flooded paddy fields of Southeast Asia.

In areas of intensive farming, where crops are harvested at least once a year and no animals browse the fields, human intervention in the form of fertilizers is important. A traditional form of fertilizer has been animal manure, or muck, made from the straw bedding of cattle that has been soaked in excreta and allowed to ferment for a period. Since the 1800s farmers also have used artificial fertilizers, at first using naturally occurring mixtures of chemicals such as chalk (supplying calcium), rock phosphates, and the natural manure known as guano. Commercial guano consists of the accumulated deposits of bird droppings and is valued for its high concentration of nitrates. Modern chemical fertilizers include one or more of three important elements: nitrogen, potassium, and phosphorus. Most nitrogenous fertilizers are produced by a technique in which nitrogen and hydrogen are combined at very high pressures in the presence of catalysts to form ammonia ($NH_3$). This can then be injected into the soil as a gas that is quickly absorbed or, more commonly, converted into solid products such as ammonium salts, urea, and nitrates, which can be used as ingredients in mixed fertilizers.

## Nutrition in Bacteria

These small organisms, popularly thought of only as sources of infection, are of vital importance in the overall life cycles of plants and animals. They commonly have to digest their food, as do larger organisms, and their cell walls do not allow the passage of large compounds. If the bacteria are in a liquid containing sugars, the sugars will diffuse through the bacterial wall and then typically be consolidated into larger molecules so that the concentration gradient will continue to promote inward diffusion. However, in order to utilize larger molecules such as starches and protein, bacteria have to excrete digestive enzymes (i.e., catalysts) into the surrounding fluid. This is obviously an expensive function for an individual organism, because much of the secreted enzymes and also the digested products may drift away from, rather than toward, the bacterial cell. However, for a cluster of thousands or millions of bacteria acting in the same way, the process is less expensive.

Bacteria vary greatly in their nutritional requirements. Some, like plants, require a source of energy such as sugars and only inorganic nutrients. Some are aerobic, meaning that they require oxygen in order to capture energy—for example, by oxidation of sugars to carbon dioxide and water. Others are anaerobic (in some cases, actually poisoned by oxygen) and require an energy source such as a sugar that they can ferment either to lactic acid or to ethanol and carbon dioxide—obtaining less energy in the process, but enough to meet their needs.

Apparently as an adaptation to many generations of living in a nutrient-rich medium, some bacteria have lost the ability to synthesize many essential compounds. For example, many of the Lactobacilli, commonly found in unsterilized milk, require essentially all the water-soluble vitamins and amino acids needed by animals. Because of this, they have been used as convenient models for assaying the value of foods as sources of particular nutrients.

## Nutrition in Animals

Simple observation reveals that the animal kingdom is dependent on plants for food. Even meat-eating, or carnivorous, animals such as the lion feed on grazing animals and thus are indirectly dependent on the plant kingdom for their survival.

## Herbivores

Plant cell walls are constructed mainly of cellulose, a material that the digestive enzymes of higher animals are unable to digest or disrupt. Because of this, even the nutritious contents of plant cells are not fully available for digestion. As an evolutionary response to this problem, many leaf eaters, or herbivores, have developed a pouch at the anterior end of the stomach, called the rumen that provides a space for the bacterial fermentation of ingested leaves. In ruminant species such as cattle and sheep, fermented material, called cud, is regurgitated from the rumen so that the animal can chew it into even smaller pieces and spread the ruminal fluid throughout the mass of ingesta. Microorganisms found in the ruminal fluid ferment cellulose to acetic acid and other short-chain fatty acids, which can then be absorbed and utilized as energy sources. Protein within the cells of the leaves is also released and degraded; some is resynthesized for digestion as microbial protein in the true stomach and small intestine. Another action of ruminal bacteria is the synthesis of some water-soluble vitamins so that, under most conditions, the host animal no longer requires them to be supplied in its food.

Because conditions in the rumen are anaerobic, another effect of ruminal fermentation is that the fatty material in the food becomes hydrogenated. Many metabolic reactions in organisms involve the removal of hydrogen atoms, and if the surplus hydrogen cannot be combined with oxygen to form water, an alternative pathway is for it to be added to unsaturated fatty acids. The result is more saturated fatty acids, which, after absorption, form deposits of harder fat. Thus, beef fat (suet) is characteristically harder at room temperature than is pork or chicken fat. Butterfat, too, is relatively saturated, being kept somewhat soft at room temperature only by the inclusion of short-chain fatty acids in the glycerol esters. This lack of the essential polyunsaturated fatty acids in ruminant fats can make them less desirable as human food.

Other herbivores make efficient use of leafy foods through hindgut fermentation. In animal species generally, the main breakdown of foods by enzymes and absorption into the bloodstream occurs in the small intestine. The main function of the large intestine is then to absorb most of the water remaining so as to conserve losses when the water supply is limited. In the "hindgut fermenters," undigested food residues undergo bacterial fermentation in the cecum, a side pocket at the distal end of the small intestine, before moving into the large intestine. In the large intestine the short-chain fatty acids produced in the cecum are absorbed and utilized. Animals in this class include horses, zebras, elephants, rhinoceroses, koalas, and rabbits.

Hindgut fermenters are somewhat less efficient than are ruminants at digesting very high-fibre foods. However, only indigestible residues are fermented in the cecum, so that hindgut fermenters do not experience the inevitable energy loss that occurs when dietary carbohydrates are fermented in the rumen. Also, the smaller bulk of the cecum allows these animals to be more athletic and better able to escape their carnivore predators.

## Carnivores

Carnivores necessarily form only a small portion of the animal kingdom, because each animal must eat a great many other animals of equivalent size in order to maintain itself over a lifetime. In addition to possessing the teeth and claws needed to kill their prey and then tear the flesh apart, carnivores have digestive enzymes that are able to break down muscle protein into amino acids, which can then diffuse through the walls of the small intestine. Therefore, carnivores have no need for any special development of the gut that allows for fermentation. Carnivores are also able to utilize animal fat. If their prey is small, they can chew and swallow bones, which serve as a source of calcium. Some carnivores, particularly cats (family *Felidae*), are obligate carnivores, meaning they cannot obtain all the nutrients that they need from the plant kingdom and bacteria. In particular, obligate carnivores lack the enzyme needed to split carotene, obtained from plants, into vitamin A. Instead, these animals obtain vitamin A from the liver of their prey. Obligate carnivores are similarly unable to synthesize some essential very-long-chain, highly unsaturated fatty acids that other animals can make from shorter fatty acids found in plants.

## Omnivores

Omnivores are miscellaneous species whose teeth and digestive systems seem designed to eat a relatively concentrated diet, since they have no large sac or chamber for the fermentation of fibrous material. They are able to chew and digest meat, though they do not have an absolute requirement for it unless there is no other practical source of vitamin $B_{12}$ (cobalamin). Humans are in this category, as are dogs, rodents, and most monkeys. All omnivores have active bacterial flora in their small cecum and large intestine and can absorb short-chain fatty acids at this point but not vitamins. Some species obtain essential vitamins by coprophagy, the eating of a proportion of their fecal pellets that contain vitamins synthesized by bacteria. Chickens, too, are omnivores. They have to swallow food without chewing it, but the food passes to an organ called the gizzard, where seeds and other foods are ground to slurry, often with the aid of swallowed stones.

## Nutrients

Some precursors (i.e., the substances from which other substances are formed) of cell materials can be synthesized by the cell from other materials, while others must be supplied in foods. All the inorganic materials required for growth, together with an assortment of organic compounds whose number may vary from 1 to 30 or more, depending on the organism, fall into the latter category. Although organisms are able to synthesize nonessential nutrients, such nutrients are frequently utilized directly if present in food, thereby saving the organism the need to expend the energy required to synthesize them.

## Inorganic Nutrients

A number of inorganic elements (minerals) are essential for the growth of living things. Boron, for example, has been demonstrated to be required for the growth of many—perhaps all—higher plants but has not been implicated as an essential element in the nutrition of either microorganisms or animals. Trace amounts of fluorine (as fluoride) are certainly beneficial, and perhaps essential, for proper tooth formation in higher animals. Similarly, iodine (as iodide) is required in animals for formation of thyroxine, the active component of an important regulatory hormone. Silicon (as silicate) is a prominent component of the outer skeletons of diatomaceous protozoans and similar organisms and is required in them for normal growth. In higher animals the requirement for silicon is much smaller. A less obvious example of a specialized mineral requirement is provided by calcium, which is required by higher animals in comparatively large amounts because it is a major component of bone and eggshells (in birds); for other organisms, calcium is an essential nutrient but only as a trace element. Mineral elements in wide variety are present in trace amounts in almost all foodstuffs. It cannot be assumed that the nonessential mineral elements play no useful role in metabolism.

Important antagonistic relationships between certain mineral nutrients also are known. A large excess of rubidium, for example, interferes with the utilization of potassium in some lactic-acid bacteria; zinc can interfere with manganese utilization in the same organism. In animal nutrition, excessive molybdenum or zinc (both of which are essential minerals) interferes with the utilization of copper, another essential mineral, and, in higher plants, excessive zinc can lead to a disorder that is known as iron chlorosis. Proper nutrient growth media for microorganisms and plants or diets for animals, therefore, require not only that the essential mineral elements be provided in sufficient amounts but also that they be used in the proper ratios to each other.

## Organic Nutrients

The organic nutrients are the necessary building blocks of various cell components that certain organisms cannot synthesize and therefore must obtain preformed. These compounds include carbohydrates, protein, and lipids. Other organic nutrients include the vitamins, which are required in small amounts, because of either the catalytic role or the regulatory role they play in metabolism.

## Carbohydrates

Quantitatively, the most important of nutrients are the carbohydrates synthesized by plants, since they provide most of the energy utilized by the animal kingdom. Mature fruit is rich in sugars that attract birds and other small animals. The seed coats in the fruit survive their rapid passage through the gut of these animals, who thus scatter widely the still viable seeds of the plant. Sucrose, in particular, also accumulates in the stems of sugarcane and in the roots of sugar beet, serving as an energy reserve for each plant; both are used for the industrial production of table sugar.

Composition of cellulose and glucose. Cellulose and glucose are examples of carbohydrates.

Dietary sugars include monosaccharides, which contain one sugar (glucose) unit, and disaccharides, which are made up of two sugar units linked together. In order to be utilized by an organism, all complex carbohydrates must be broken down into simple sugars, which, in most cases, are rapidly digested and absorbed. For example, even the freely soluble disaccharide sucrose must first be hydrolyzed to glucose and fructose by a specific enzyme, sucrase. Newborn piglets do not secrete this enzyme and therefore cannot make use of sucrose. Conversely, the disaccharide lactose is rapidly hydrolyzed by newborn animals, but most species—even some humans—stop secreting the enzyme lactase after weaning. This is understandable since lactose occurs naturally only in milk, which an animal usually will not encounter again after its suckling period.

The major storage carbohydrate in plant seeds, starch is a polysaccharide, formed from the condensation of several glucose units, primarily through linkages that are rapidly broken down by digestive enzymes in microorganisms as well as in higher animals. However, different plant starches vary in the cross-linkages between these basic chains, and this variation can result in more compact molecules that are resistant to digestion. One of the major effects of cooking is that starch granules swell with absorbed water and become more easily digestible. Surprisingly, even members of the cat family, which would not encounter starch in their natural carnivorous diet, can utilize it quite efficiently when it is finely ground. Commercial dry cat foods may contain 20 percent or more starch.

Plant cell walls are constructed principally from cellulose. Cellulose is like starch in that it is made from condensed glucose units, but a different type of linkage between these units allows the chains to lie in flat planes, and vertebrates have no enzymes to digest these linkages. However, herbivorous species have gastrointestinal systems that allow for the bacterial fermentation of cellulose either in a fore-stomach (rumen) or hindgut, which enables the animals to benefit from the metabolites of cellulose, principally short-chain fatty acids. Other polysaccharides in plant cell walls include pectins and hemicelluloses, which give a mixture of sugars, such as xylose and arabinose, upon hydrolysis. These sugars also are fermented by bacteria but are not broken down and digested by animal enzymes. Rigid plant structures contain lignin, a phenolic polymer that is impervious to digestion by both animals and bacteria. Considered together, these materials make up what is called dietary fibre.

## Lipids (Fats and Oils)

Another form in which some plants store energy in their seeds is fat, commonly called oil in its liquid form. In animals, fats form the only large-scale energy store. Fats are a more concentrated energy source than carbohydrates; oxidation yields roughly nine and four kilocalories of energy per gram, respectively.

A fat consists of three fatty acids (i.e., a hydrocarbon chain with a carboxylic acid group at one end) attached to a glycerol backbone. The physical properties of fats depend on the fatty acids that they contain. All fats are liquid when present in living tissues. The fats of warm-blooded animals can, of course, have a higher freezing point than that of cold-blooded animals such as fish. Plants that survive frosts must have a particularly low freezing point. In general, organisms lay down fat that has little or no excess of liquidity; that is, it has a freezing point near the maximum consistent with the organism's viability.

Fatty acids differ from one another in two ways: Chain length and saturation. Chain length varies from 4 to 22 carbons, with most fatty acids having 16 or 18 carbons. The relatively low freezing point of a cow's butterfat results from its content of the 4-carbon short-chain fatty acid butyric acid; the longer the saturated chains, the higher the freezing point of the acids themselves and of the fat containing them. However, a greater effect of liquidity comes from the introduction of un-saturated (double) bonds in the chains. More than one double bond (polyunsaturation) makes it more difficult for fats to remain solid at room temperature.

Animals generally either store absorbed fatty acids or oxidize them immediately as a source of en-ergy. Particular fatty acids are needed for the production of phospholipids, which form an essential portion of cell membranes and nerve fibres, and for the synthesis of certain hormones. Animals can synthesize their own fat from an excess of absorbed sugars, but they are limited in their ability to synthesize essential polyunsaturated fatty acids such as linoleic acid and linolenic acid. Thus, fatty acids are not just an alternative energy source—they are a vital dietary ingredient. The main vegetable oils are good sources of linoleic acid, and most of these also contain a smaller propor-tion of linolenic acid. Cats have lost one of the principal enzymes used by other animals to convert linoleic acid to arachidonic acid, which is needed for the synthesis of prostaglandins and other hormones. Since arachidonic acid is not found in plants, cats are obligate carnivores, meaning that under natural conditions they must eat animal tissue in order to survive and reproduce.

## Proteins

The main organic material in the working tissue of both plants and animals is protein, large mol-ecules containing chains of condensed units of some 20 different amino acids. In animals, protein food is digested to free amino acids before entering the bloodstream. Plants can synthesize their own amino acids, which are required for protein production, provided they have a source of nitrate or other simple nitrogenous compounds and sulfur, needed for the synthesis of cysteine and me-thionine. Animals can also synthesize some amino acids from ammonium ions and carbohydrate metabolites; however, others cannot be synthesized and are therefore dietary essentials. Two ami-no acids, cysteine and tyrosine, can be synthesized only by metabolism of the essential amino acids methionine and phenylalanine, respectively. Bacteria living in the rumen of ruminant animals can synthesize all the amino acids commonly present in protein, and the true stomach of the ruminant will continue to receive microbial protein of reasonably good quality for digestion.

Animals need protein to grow. This requirement is roughly proportional to the growth rate and is reflected in the protein content of the milk secreted during the suckling period. For example, a piglet doubles its birth weight in 18 days, and sow's milk has protein at a level supplying 25 percent of the total energy. In contrast, humans take approximately 180 days to double their birth weight, and breast milk contains protein at a level equivalent to only about 8 percent of the total energy. Young animals fed experimental diets completely lacking one essential amino acid all exhibit an immediate cessation of growth.

Adults, too, require protein in fairly large amounts, more than would be needed to replace the small amount of protein lost by the body through urine, feces, and shed hair and skin. It is true that animal tissues are continually "turning over" their proteins—i.e., hydrolyzing and re-synthesizing them—but this does not explain the additional protein requirement, since the amino acids released are available for reuse. It appears, however, that the enzymes available to metabolize excess amino acids do not inactivate completely when the body is short of protein but instead remain at an "idling" rate. Normally, this is not a disadvantage, since the diets of adult animals, including humans, contain more protein than is required to balance the idling losses. It also appears that, in the course of evolution, the idling rates have become roughly adjusted to the normal protein intake. Thus, adult rodents living on a range of foods—some quite low in protein—need no more than 5 percent of their energy in the form of protein. In contrast, cats, whose ancestral carnivorous diet was much higher in protein, need some 20 percent in their diet to balance minimal losses.

## Vitamins

Vitamins may be defined as organic substances that play a required catalytic role within the cell (usually as components of coenzymes or other groups associated with enzymes) and must be obtained in small amounts through the diet. Vitamin requirements are specific for each organism, and their deficiency may cause disease. Vitamin deficiencies in young animals usually result in growth failure, various symptoms whose nature depends on the vitamin, and eventual death.

Although a vitamin is usually defined as an organic chemical which an animal or human must obtain from the diet in very small amounts, this is not entirely true. Vitamin A does not occur in the plant kingdom, but the pigment carotene is universally present in green plants, and most animals can split a molecule of carotene into two molecules of vitamin A. The exceptions are cats and probably other carnivores, which under natural conditions have to obtain the preformed vitamin by consuming the tissues of other animals. Niacin, too, is not an absolute requirement, since most animals (cats again being an exception) can synthesize it from the amino acid tryptophan if the latter is present in excess of its use for protein synthesis.

Vitamin D is not a true vitamin: Most species do not need it in their diet, because they obtain an adequate supply through the exposure of skin to sunlight, which converts a sterol present in dermal tissue to vitamin D. The vitamin is subsequently metabolized to form a hormone that acts to control the absorption and utilization of calcium and phosphate. Animals such as rodents, which normally have little exposure to sunlight and search for food mostly at night, appear to have evolved so as to be independent of vitamin D so long as their intakes of calcium and phosphate are well-balanced.

Vitamin C (ascorbic acid) is an essential chemical in the tissues of all species, but most can make it for themselves, so that for them it is not a vitamin. Presumably, species that cannot synthesize vitamin C—they include humans, guinea pigs, and fruit-eating bats—had ancestors that lost the ability at a time when their diet was rich in ascorbic acid.

Bacteria vary greatly in their need for vitamins. Many are entirely independent of outside sources, but at the other extreme some of the strains of bacteria found in milk (i.e., Lactobacillus) have lost the ability to synthesize the B vitamins that they need. This property has made them useful for assaying extracts of foods for their vitamin B content. Indeed, many vitamins of this group were first discovered as growth factors for bacteria before being tested with animals and humans. The mixed bacterial flora in the guts of animals are, on balance, synthesizers of the B vitamins. Consequently, ruminant animals do not have to obtain them from an external source. On the other hand, the ability of hindgut fermenters to absorb vitamins from their large intestine is uncertain. Rats and rabbits, whose nutritional needs have been studied intensively, have both been found to engage in coprophagy, the eating of fecal pellets that are vitamin-rich as a result of bacterial fermentation in the hindgut.

For one B vitamin—cobalamin, or vitamin $B_{12}$—bacterial fermentation is the only source, though it can be obtained indirectly from the tissues or milk of animals that have obtained it themselves from bacteria. The generalization that "the animal kingdom lives on the plant kingdom" is therefore not the whole truth, because animals rely partly on bacteria for this one micronutrient.

## Interdependency of Nutritional Requirements

The effects of one mineral nutrient in reducing or increasing the requirement for another have been mentioned previously. Similar relationships occur among organic nutrients and originate for several reasons.

## Competition for Sites of Absorption by the Cell

Since absorption of nutrients frequently occurs by way of active transport within cell membranes, an excess of one nutrient (A) may inhibit absorption of a second nutrient (B), if they share the same absorption pathway. In such cases, the apparent requirement for nutrient B increases; B, however, can sometimes be supplied in an alternate form that is able to enter the cell by a different route. Many examples of amino acid antagonism, in which inhibition of growth by one amino acid is counteracted by another amino acid, are best explained by this mechanism. For example, under some conditions Lactobacillus casei requires both D- and L-alanine, which differ from each other only in the position of the amino, or $NH_2$, group in the molecule, and the two forms of this amino acid share the same absorption pathway. Excess D-alanine inhibits growth of this species, but the inhibition can be alleviated either by supplying additional L-alanine or, more effectively, by supplying peptides of L-alanine. The peptides enter the cell by a pathway different from that of the two forms of alanine and, after they are in the cell, can be broken down to form L-alanine. Relationships of this type provide one explanation for the fact that peptides are frequently more effective than amino acids in promoting growth of bacteria.

## Competition for Sites of Utilization within the Cell

This phenomenon is similar to that regarding competition for absorption sites, but it occurs inside the cell and only between structurally similar nutrients (e.g., leucine and valine; serine and threonine).

## Precursor-product Relationships

The requirement of rats and humans for the essential amino acids phenylalanine and methionine is substantially reduced if tyrosine, which is formed from phenylalanine, or cysteine, which is formed from methionine, is added to the diet. These relationships are explained by the fact that tyrosine and cysteine are synthesized in animals from phenylalanine and methionine, respectively. When the former (product) amino acids are supplied preformed, the latter (precursor) amino acids are required in smaller amounts. Several instances of the sparing of one nutrient by another because they have similar precursor-product relationships have been identified in other organisms.

## Changes in Metabolic Pathways within the Cell

Rats fed diets containing large amounts of fat require substantially less thiamin (vitamin $B_1$) than do those fed diets high in carbohydrate. The utilization of carbohydrate as an energy source (i.e., for ATP formation) is known to involve an important thiamin-dependent step, which is bypassed when fat is used as an energy source, and it is assumed that the lessened requirement for thiamin results from the change in metabolic pathways.

## Syntrophism

Since the nutritional requirements and metabolic activities of organisms differ, it is clear that two or more different organisms growing relatedly may produce different overall changes in the environment. A rough example is provided by a balanced aquarium, in which aquatic plants utilize light and the waste products of animals—e.g., carbon dioxide, water, ammonia—to synthesize cell materials and generate oxygen, which in turn provide the materials necessary for animal growth. Such relationships are common among microorganisms; i.e., intermediate or end products of metabolism of one organism may provide essential nutrients for another. The mixed populations that result in nature provide examples of this phenomenon, which is called syntrophism; in some instances, the relationship may be so close as to constitute nutritional symbiosis, or mutualism. Several examples of this phenomenon have been found among thiamin-requiring yeasts and fungi, certain of which (group A) synthesized the thiazole component of thiamin molecule but require the pyrimidine portion preformed; for a second group (group B), the relationship is reversed. When group A and group B are grown together in a thiamin-free medium, both types of organisms survive, since each organism synthesizes the growth factor required by its partner; neither organism grows alone under these same conditions. Thus, two or more types of microorganisms frequently grow in situations in which only one species would not.

Such nutritional interrelationships may explain the fact that the nutritionally demanding lactic-acid bacteria are able to coexist with the nutritionally nondemanding coliform bacteria in the intestinal tracts of animals. It is known that the bacterial flora of the intestinal tract synthesize sufficient amounts of certain vitamins (e.g., vitamin K, folic acid) so that detection of deficiency symptoms in rats requires special measures, and the role of rumen bacteria in ruminant animals (e.g., cows, sheep) in rendering otherwise indigestible cellulose and other materials available to the host animal is well-known. These few examples indicate that syntrophic interrelationships are widespread in nature and may contribute substantially to the nutrition of a wide variety of species.

# Human Nutrition

Human nutrition is the process by which substances in food are transformed into body tissues and provide energy for the full range of physical and mental activities that make up human life.

The study of human nutrition is interdisciplinary in character, involving not only physiology, biochemistry, and molecular biology but also fields such as psychology and anthropology, which explore the influence of attitudes, beliefs, preferences, and cultural traditions on food choices. Human nutrition further touches on economics and political science as the world community recognizes and responds to the suffering and death caused by malnutrition. The ultimate goal of nutritional science is to promote optimal health and reduce the risk of chronic diseases such as cardiovascular disease and cancer as well as to prevent classic nutritional deficiency diseases such as kwashiorkor and pellagra.

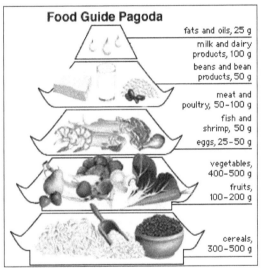

**Food Guide Pagoda**

fats and oils, 25 g
milk and dairy products, 100 g
beans and bean products, 50 g
meat and poultry, 50–100 g
fish and shrimp, 50 g
eggs, 25–50 g
vegetables, 400–500 g
fruits, 100–200 g
cereals, 300–500 g

In a style that reflects the culinary traditions of China, the Food Guide Pagoda recommends a liberal daily intake of grain products (represented by the wide base of the pagoda) and a sparing intake of fats and oils (represented by the tip of the structure).

## Utilization of Food by the Body

## Calories and Kilocalories: Energy Supply

The human body can be thought of as an engine that releases the energy present in the foods that it digests. This energy is utilized partly for the mechanical work performed by the muscles and in the secretory processes and partly for the work necessary to maintain the body's structure and functions. The performance of work is associated with the production of heat; heat loss is controlled so as to keep body temperature within a narrow range. Unlike other engines, however, the human body is continually breaking down (catabolizing) and building up (anabolizing) its component parts. Foods supply nutrients essential to the manufacture of the new material and provide energy needed for the chemical reactions involved.

Carbohydrate, fat, and protein are, to a large extent, interchangeable as sources of energy. Typically, the energy provided by food is measured in kilocalories, or Calories. One kilocalorie is equal to

1,000 gram-calories (or small calories), a measure of heat energy. However, in common parlance, kilocalories are referred to as "calories." In other words, a 2,000-calorie diet actually has 2,000 kilocalories of potential energy. One kilocalorie is the amount of heat energy required to raise one kilogram of water from 14.5 to 15.5 °C at one atmosphere of pressure. Another unit of energy widely used is the joule, which measures energy in terms of mechanical work. One joule is the energy expended when one kilogram is moved a distance of one metre by a force of one newton. The relatively higher levels of energy in human nutrition are more likely to be measured in kilojoules (1 kilojoule = $10^3$ joules) or megajoules (1 megajoule = $10^6$ joules). One kilocalorie is equivalent to 4.184 kilojoules.

The energy present in food can be determined directly by measuring the output of heat when the food is burned (oxidized) in a bomb calorimeter. However, the human body is not as efficient as a calorimeter, and some potential energy is lost during digestion and metabolism. Corrected physiological values for the heats of combustion of the three energy-yielding nutrients, rounded to whole numbers, are as follows: carbohydrate, 4 kilocalories (17 kilojoules) per gram; protein, 4 kilocalories (17 kilojoules) per gram; and fat, 9 kilocalories (38 kilojoules) per gram. Beverage alcohol (ethyl alcohol) also yields energy—7 kilocalories (29 kilojoules) per gram—although it is not essential in the diet. Vitamins, minerals, water, and other food constituents have no energy value, although many of them participate in energy-releasing processes in the body.

The energy provided by a well-digested food can be estimated if the gram amounts of energy-yielding substances (non-fibre carbohydrate, fat, protein, and alcohol) in that food are known. For example, a slice of white bread containing 12 grams of carbohydrate, 2 grams of protein, and 1 gram of fat supplies 67 kilocalories (280 kilojoules) of energy. Food composition tables and food labels provide useful data for evaluating energy and nutrient intake of an individual diet. Most foods provide a mixture of energy-supplying nutrients, along with vitamins, minerals, water, and other substances. Two notable exceptions are table sugar and vegetable oil, which are virtually pure carbohydrate (sucrose) and fat, respectively.

Throughout most of the world, protein supplies between 8 and 16 percent of the energy in the diet, although there are wide variations in the proportions of fat and carbohydrate in different populations. In more prosperous communities about 12 to 15 percent of energy is typically derived from protein, 30 to 40 percent from fat, and 50 to 60 percent from carbohydrate. On the other hand, in many poorer agricultural societies, where cereals comprise the bulk of the diet, carbohydrate provides an even larger percentage of energy, with protein and fat providing less. The human body is remarkably adaptable and can survive, and even thrive, on widely divergent diets. However, different dietary patterns are associated with particular health consequences.

## BMR and REE: Energy Balance

Energy is needed not only when a person is physically active but even when the body is lying motionless. Depending on an individual's level of physical activity, between 50 and 80 percent of the energy expended each day is devoted to basic metabolic processes (basal metabolism), which enable the body to stay warm, breathe, pump blood, and conduct numerous physiological and biosynthetic activities, including synthesis of new tissue in growing children and in pregnant and lactating women. Digestion and subsequent processing of food by the body also uses energy and produces heat. This phenomenon, known as the thermic effect of food (or diet-induced thermogenesis), accounts for about 10 percent of daily energy expenditure, varying somewhat with the composition of the diet and prior dietary practices. Adaptive thermogenesis, another small but important component of energy expenditure, reflects alterations in metabolism due to changes in ambient temperature, hormone production, emotional stress, or other factors. Finally, the most variable component in energy expenditure is physical activity, which includes exercise and other voluntary activities as well as involuntary activities such as fidgeting, shivering, and maintaining posture. Physical activity accounts for 20 to 40 percent of the total energy expenditure, even less in a very sedentary person and more in someone who is extremely active.

Basal or resting energy expenditure is correlated primarily with lean body mass (fat-free mass and essential fat, excluding storage fat), which is the metabolically active tissue in the body. At rest, organs such as the liver, brain, heart, and kidney have the highest metabolic activity and, therefore, the highest need for energy, while muscle and bone require less energy and body fat even less. Besides body composition, other factors affecting basal metabolism include age, sex, body temperature, and thyroid hormone levels.

The basal metabolic rate (BMR), a precisely defined measure of the energy expenditure necessary to support life, is determined under controlled and standardized conditions—shortly after awakening in the morning, at least 12 hours after the last meal, and with a comfortable room temperature. Because of practical considerations, the BMR is rarely measured; the resting energy expenditure (REE) is determined under less stringent conditions, with the individual resting comfortably about 2 to 4 hours after a meal. In practice, the BMR and REE differ by no more than 10 percent—the REE is usually slightly higher—and the terms are used interchangeably.

Energy expenditure can be assessed by direct calorimetry, or measurement of heat dissipated from the body, which employs apparatuses such as water-cooled garments or insulated chambers large enough to accommodate a person. However, energy expenditure is usually measured by the less cumbersome techniques of indirect calorimetry, in which heat produced by the body is calculated from measurements of oxygen inhaled, carbon dioxide exhaled, and urinary nitrogen excreted. The BMR (in kilocalories per day) can be roughly estimated using the following formula: BMR = $70 \times$ (body weight in kilograms)$^{3/4}$.

The energy costs of various activities have been measured. While resting may require as little as 1 kilocalorie per minute, strenuous work may demand 10 times that much. Mental activity, though it may seem taxing, has no appreciable effect on energy requirement. A 70-kg (154-pound) man, whose REE over the course of a day might be 1,750 kilocalories, could expend a total of 2,400 kilocalories on a very sedentary day and up to 4,000 kilocalories on a very active day. A 55-kg (121-pound) woman, whose daily resting energy expenditure might be 1,350 kilocalories, could use from 1,850 to more than 3,000 total kilocalories, depending on level of activity.

Table: Approximate energy expenditure for activity levels.

| Activity category | Energy as multiple of resting energy expenditure (ree) | kilocalories per minute |
|---|---|---|
| Resting (sleeping, reclining). | Ree × 1.0 | 1–1.2 |
| Very light (driving, typing, cooking). | Ree × 1.5 | up to 2.5 |
| Light (walking on a level surface at 4 to 5 km/hr [2.5 to 3 mph], golf and table tennis). | Ree × 2.5 | 2.5–4.9 |

| Moderate (walking 5.5 to 6.5 km/hr [3.5 to 4 mph], carrying a load, cycling, tennis, skiing, dancing). | Ree × 5.0 | 5.0–7.4 |
|---|---|---|
| Heavy (walking uphill with a load, basketball, climbing, football, soccer). | Ree × 7.0 | 7.5–12.0 |

The law of conservation of energy applies: If one takes in more energy than is expended, over time one will gain weight; insufficient energy intake results in weight loss, as the body taps its energy stores to provide for immediate needs. Excess food energy is stored in small amounts as glycogen, a short-term storage form of carbohydrate in muscle and liver, and as fat, the body's main energy reserve found in adipose tissue. Adipose tissue is mostly fat (about 87 percent), but it also contains some protein and water. In order to lose 454 grams (one pound) of adipose tissue, an energy deficit of about 3,500 kilocalories (14.6 megajoules) is required.

## Body Mass, Body Fat and Body Water

The human body consists of materials similar to those found in foods; however, the relative proportions differ, according to genetic dictates as well as to the unique life experience of the individual. The body of a healthy lean man is composed of roughly 62 percent water, 16 percent fat, 16 percent protein, 6 percent minerals, and less than 1 percent carbohydrate, along with very small amounts of vitamins and other miscellaneous substances. Females usually carry more fat (about 22 percent in a healthy lean woman) and slightly less of the other components than do males of comparable weight.

The body's different compartments—lean body mass, body fat and body water—are constantly adjusting to changes in the internal and external environment so that a state of dynamic equilibrium (homeostasis) is maintained. Tissues in the body are continuously being broken down (catabolism) and built up (anabolism) at varying rates. For example, the epithelial cells lining the digestive tract are replaced at a dizzying speed of every three or four days, while the life span of red blood cells is 120 days, and connective tissue is renewed over the course of several years.

Although estimates of the percentage of body fat can be made by direct inspection, this approach is imprecise. Body fat can be measured indirectly using fairly precise but costly methods, such as underwater weighing, total body potassium counting, and dual-energy X-ray absorptiometry (DXA). However, more practical, albeit less accurate, methods are often used, such as anthropometry, in which subcutaneous fat at various sites is measured using skinfold calipers; bioelectrical impedance, in which resistance to a low-intensity electrical current is used to estimate body fat; and near infrared interactance, in which an infrared light aimed at the biceps is used to assess fat and protein interaction. Direct measurement of the body's various compartments can only be performed on cadavers.

The composition of the body tends to change in somewhat predictable ways over the course of a lifetime—during the growing years, in pregnancy and lactation, and as one ages—with corresponding changes in nutrient needs during different phases of the life cycle. Regular physical exercise can help attenuate the age-related loss of lean tissue and increase in body fat.

## Essential Nutrients

The six classes of nutrients found in foods are carbohydrates, lipids (mostly fats and oils), proteins, vitamins, minerals, and water. Carbohydrates, lipids, and proteins constitute the bulk of the diet, amounting together to about 500 grams (just over one pound) per day in actual weight. These macronutrients provide raw materials for tissue building and maintenance as well as fuel to run the myriad of physiological and metabolic activities that sustain life. In contrast are the micronutrients, which are not themselves energy sources but facilitate metabolic processes throughout the body: vitamins, of which humans need about 300 milligrams per day in the diet, and minerals, of which about 20 grams per day are needed. The last nutrient category is water, which provides the medium in which all the body's metabolic processes occur.

A nutrient is considered "essential" if it must be taken in from outside the body—in most cases, from food. Although they are separated into categories for purposes of discussion, one should keep in mind that nutrients work in collaboration with each other in the body, not as isolated entities.

## Carbohydrates

Carbohydrates, which are composed of carbon, hydrogen, and oxygen, are the major supplier of energy to the body, providing 4 kilocalories per gram. In most carbohydrates, the elements hydrogen and oxygen are present in the same 2:1 ratio as in water, thus "carbo" (for carbon) and "hydrate" (for water).

## Glucose

The simple carbohydrate glucose is the principal fuel used by the brain and nervous system and by red blood cells. Muscle and other body cells can also use glucose for energy, although fat is often used for this purpose. Because a steady supply of glucose is so critical to cells, blood glucose is maintained within a relatively narrow range through the action of various hormones, mainly insulin, which directs the flow of glucose into cells, and glucagon and epinephrine, which retrieve glucose from storage. The body stores a small amount of glucose as glycogen, a complex branched form of carbohydrate, in liver and muscle tissue, and this can be broken down to glucose and used as an energy source during short periods (a few hours) of fasting or during times of intense physical activity or stress. If blood glucose falls below normal (hypoglycemia), weakness and dizziness may result. Elevated blood glucose (hyperglycemia), as can occur in diabetes, is also dangerous and cannot be left untreated.

Glucose can be made in the body from most types of carbohydrate and from protein, although protein is usually an expensive source of energy. Some minimal amount of carbohydrate is required in the diet—at least 50 to 100 grams a day. This not only spares protein but also ensures that fats are completely metabolized and prevents a condition known as ketosis, the accumulation of products of fat breakdown, called ketones, in the body. Although there are great variations in the quantity and type of carbohydrates eaten throughout the world, most diets contain more than enough.

## Other Sugars and Starch

The simplest carbohydrates are sugars, which give many foods their sweet taste but at the same time provide food for bacteria in the mouth, thus contributing to dental decay. Sugars in the diet are monosaccharides, which contain one sugar or saccharide unit, and disaccharides, which contain two saccharide units linked together. Monosaccharides of nutritional importance are glucose, fructose, and galactose; disaccharides include sucrose (table sugar), lactose (milk sugar), and maltose. A slightly more complex type of carbohydrate is the oligosaccharide (e.g., raffinose and stachyose), which contains three to 10 saccharide units; these compounds, which are found in beans and other legumes and cannot be digested well by humans, account for the gas-producing effects of these foods. Larger and more complex storage forms of carbohydrate are the polysaccharides, which consist of long chains of glucose units. Starch, the most important polysaccharide in the human diet—found in grains, legumes, potatoes, and other vegetables—is made up of mainly straight glucose chains (amylose) or mainly branching chains (amylopectin). Finally, nondigestible polysaccharides known as dietary fibre are found in plant foods such as grains, fruits, vegetables, legumes, seeds, and nuts.

In order to be utilized by the body, all complex carbohydrates must be broken down into simple sugars, which, in turn, must be broken down into monosaccharides—a feat, accomplished by enzymes, that starts in the mouth and ends in the small intestine, where most absorption takes place. Each dissacharide is split into single units by a specific enzyme; for example, the enzyme lactase breaks down lactose into its constituent monosaccharides, glucose and galactose. In much of the world's population, lactase activity declines during childhood and adolescence, which leads to an inability to digest lactose adequately. This inherited trait, called lactose intolerance, results in gastrointestinal discomfort and diarrhea if too much lactose is consumed. Those who have retained the ability to digest dairy products efficiently in adulthood are primarily of northern European ancestry.

## Dietary Fibre

Dietary fibre, the structural parts of plants, cannot be digested by the human intestine because the necessary enzymes are lacking. Even though these nondigestible compounds pass through the gut unchanged (except for a small percentage that is fermented by bacteria in the large intestine), they nevertheless contribute to good health. Insoluble fibre does not dissolve in water and provides bulk, or roughage, that helps with bowel function (regularity) and accelerates the exit from the body of potentially carcinogenic or otherwise harmful substances in food. Types of insoluble fibre are cellulose, most hemicelluloses, and lignin (a phenolic polymer, not a carbohydrate). Major food sources of insoluble fibre are whole grain breads and cereals, wheat bran, and vegetables. Soluble fibre, which dissolves or swells in water, slows down the transit time of food through the gut (an undesirable effect) but also helps lower blood cholesterol levels (a desirable effect). Types of soluble fibre are gums, pectins, some hemicelluloses, and mucilages; fruits (especially citrus fruits and apples), oats, barley, and legumes are major food sources. Both soluble and insoluble fibre help delay glucose absorption, thus ensuring a slower and more even supply of blood glucose. Dietary fibre is thought to provide important protection against some gastrointestinal diseases and to reduce the risk of other chronic diseases as well.

## Lipids

Lipids also contain carbon, hydrogen, and oxygen but in a different configuration, having considerably fewer oxygen atoms than are found in carbohydrates. Lipids are soluble in organic solvents (such as acetone or ether) and insoluble in water, a property that is readily seen when an oil-and-vinegar salad dressing separates quickly upon standing. The lipids of nutritional importance are triglycerides (fats and oils), phospholipids (e.g., lecithin), and sterols (e.g., cholesterol). Lipids in the diet transport the four fat-soluble vitamins (vitamins A, D, E, and K) and assist in their absorption in the small intestine. They also carry with them substances that impart sensory appeal and palatability to food and provide satiety value, the feeling of being full and satisfied after eating a meal. Fats in the diet are a more concentrated form of energy than carbohydrates and have an energy yield of 9 kilocalories per gram. Adipose (fatty) tissue in the fat depots of the body serves as an energy reserve as well as helping to insulate the body and cushion the internal organs.

## Triglycerides

The major lipids in food and stored in the body as fat are the triglycerides, which consist of three fatty acids attached to a backbone of glycerol (an alcohol). Fatty acids are essentially hydrocarbon chains with a carboxylic acid group (COOH) at one end, the alpha ($\alpha$) end, and a methyl group ($CH_3$) at the other, omega ($\omega$), end. They are classified as saturated or unsaturated according to their chemical structure. A point of unsaturation indicates a double bond between two carbon atoms, rather than the full complement of hydrogen atoms that is present in saturated fatty acids. A monounsaturated fatty acid has one point of unsaturation, while a polyunsaturated fatty acid has two or more.

Fatty acids found in the human diet and in body tissues range from a chain length of 4 carbons to 22 or more, each chain having an even number of carbon atoms. Of particular importance for humans are the 18-carbon polyunsaturated fatty acids alpha-linolenic acid (an omega-3 fatty acid) and linoleic acid (an omega-6 fatty acid); these are known as essential fatty acids because they are required in small amounts in the diet. The omega designations (also referred to as n-3 and n-6) indicate the location of the first double bond from the methyl end of the fatty acid. Other fatty acids can be synthesized in the body and are therefore not essential in the diet. About a tablespoon daily of an ordinary vegetable oil such as safflower or corn oil or a varied diet that includes grains, nuts, seeds, and vegetables can fulfill the essential fatty acid requirement. Essential fatty acids are needed for the formation of cell membranes and the synthesis of hormone-like compounds called eicosanoids (e.g., prostaglandins, thromboxanes, and leukotrienes), which are important regulators of blood pressure, blood clotting, and the immune response. The consumption of fish once or twice a week provides an additional source of omega-3 fatty acids that appears to be healthful.

A fat consisting largely of saturated fatty acids, especially long-chain fatty acids, tends to be solid at room temperature; if unsaturated fatty acids predominate, the fat is liquid at room temperature. Fats and oils usually contain mixtures of fatty acids, although the type of fatty acid in greatest concentration typically gives the food its characteristics. Butter and other animal fats are primarily saturated; olive and canola oils, monounsaturated; and fish, corn, safflower, soybean, and sunflower oils, polyunsaturated. Although plant oils tend to be largely unsaturated, there are notable exceptions, such as coconut fat, which is highly saturated but nevertheless semiliquid at room temperature because its fatty acids are of medium chain length (8 to 14 carbons long).

Saturated fats tend to be more stable than unsaturated ones. The food industry takes advantage of this property during hydrogenation, in which hydrogen molecules are added to a point of unsaturation, thereby making the fatty acid more stable and resistant to rancidity (oxidation) as well as more solid and spreadable (as in margarine). However, a result of the hydrogenation process is a change in the shape of some unsaturated fatty acids from a configuration known as cis to that known as trans. Trans-fatty acids, which behave more like saturated fatty acids, may also have undesirable health consequences.

## Phospholipids

A phospholipid is similar to a triglyceride except that it contains a phosphate group and a nitrogen-containing compound such as choline instead of one of the fatty acids. In food, phospholipids are natural emulsifiers, allowing fat and water to mix, and they are used as food additives for this purpose. In the body, phospholipids allow fats to be suspended in fluids such as blood, and they enable lipids to move across cell membranes from one watery compartment to another. The phospholipid lecithin is plentiful in foods such as egg yolks, liver, wheat germ, and peanuts. However, the liver is able to synthesize all the lecithin the body needs if sufficient choline is present in the diet.

## Sterols

Sterols are unique among lipids in that they have a multiple-ring structure. The well-known sterol cholesterol is found only in foods of animal origin—meat, egg yolk, fish, poultry, and dairy products. Organ meats (e.g., liver, kidney) and egg yolks have the most cholesterol, while muscle meats and cheeses have less. There are a number of sterols in shellfish but not as much cholesterol as was once thought. Cholesterol is essential to the structure of cell membranes and is also used to make other important sterols in the body, among them the sex hormones, adrenal hormones, bile acids, and vitamin D. However, cholesterol can be synthesized in the liver, so there is no need to consume it in the diet.

Cholesterol-containing deposits may build up in the walls of arteries, leading to a condition known as atherosclerosis, which contributes to myocardial infarction (heart attack) and stroke. Furthermore, because elevated levels of blood cholesterol, especially the form known as low-density lipoprotein (LDL) cholesterol, have been associated with an increased risk of cardiovascular disease, a limited intake of saturated fat—particularly medium-chain saturated fatty acids, which act to raise LDL cholesterol levels—is advised. Trans-fatty acids also raise LDL cholesterol, while monounsaturated and polyunsaturated (cis) fats tend to lower LDL cholesterol levels. Because of the body's feedback mechanisms, dietary cholesterol has only a minor influence on blood cholesterol in most people; however, since some individuals respond strongly to cholesterol in the diet, a restricted intake is often advised, especially for those at risk of heart disease.

## Proteins

Proteins, like carbohydrates and fats, contain carbon, hydrogen, and oxygen, but they also contain nitrogen, a component of the amino chemical group ($NH_2$), and in some cases sulfur. Proteins serve as the basic structural material of the body as well as being biochemical catalysts and regulators of genes. Aside from water, protein constitutes the major part of muscles, bones, internal organs, and the skin, nails, and hair. Protein is also an important part of cell membranes and blood (e.g., hemoglobin). Enzymes, which catalyze chemical reactions in the body, are also protein, as are antibodies, collagen in connective tissue, and many hormones, such as insulin.

Tissues throughout the body require ongoing repair and replacement, and thus the body's protein is turning over constantly, being broken down and then resynthesized as needed. Tissue proteins are in a dynamic equilibrium with proteins in the blood, with input from proteins in the diet and losses through urine, feces, and skin. In a healthy adult, adjustments are made so that the amount of protein lost is in balance with the amount of protein ingested. However, during periods of rapid growth, pregnancy and lactation, or recuperation after illness or depletion, the body is in positive nitrogen balance, as more protein is being retained than excreted. The opposite is true during illness or wasting, when there is negative nitrogen balance as more tissue is being broken down than synthesized.

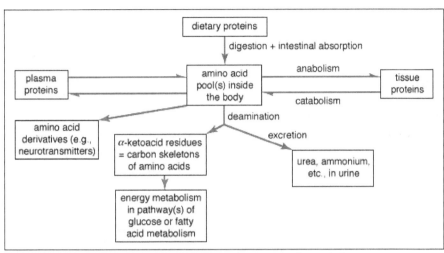

General scheme of protein and amino acid metabolism.

## Amino Acids

The proteins in food—such as albumin in egg white, casein in dairy products, and gluten in wheat—are broken down during digestion into constituent amino acids, which, when absorbed, contribute to the body's metabolic pool. Amino acids are then joined via peptide linkages to assemble specific proteins, as directed by the genetic material and in response to the body's needs at the time. Each gene makes one or more proteins, each with a unique sequence of amino acids and precise three-dimensional configuration. Amino acids are also required for the synthesis of other important nonprotein compounds, such as peptide hormones, some neurotransmitters, and creatine.

Food contains approximately 20 common amino acids, 9 of which are considered essential, or indispensable, for humans; i.e., they cannot be synthesized by the body or cannot be synthesized in sufficient quantities and therefore must be taken in the diet. The essential amino acids for humans are histidine, isoleucine, leucine, lysine, methionine, phenylalanine, threonine, tryptophan, and valine. Conditionally indispensable amino acids include arginine, cysteine, and tyrosine, which may need to be provided under special circumstances, such as in premature infants or in people with liver disease, because of impaired conversion from precursors.

The relative proportions of different amino acids vary from food to food. Foods of animal origin—meat, fish, eggs, and dairy products—are sources of good quality, or complete, protein; i.e., their essential amino acid patterns are similar to human needs for protein. (Gelatin, which lacks the amino acid tryptophan, is an exception). Individual foods of plant origin, with the exception of soybeans, are lower quality, or incomplete, protein sources. Lysine, methionine, and tryptophan are the primary limiting amino acids; i.e., they are in smallest supply and therefore limit the amount of protein that can be synthesized. However, a varied vegetarian diet can readily fulfill human protein requirements if the protein-containing foods are balanced such that their essential amino acids complement each other. For example, legumes such as beans are high in lysine and low in methionine, while grains have complementary strengths and weaknesses. Thus, if beans and rice are eaten over the course of a day, their joint amino acid patterns will supplement each other and provide a higher quality protein than would either food alone. Traditional food patterns in native cultures have made good use of protein complementarity. However, careful balancing of plant proteins is necessary only for those whose protein intake is marginal or inadequate. In affluent populations, where protein intake is greatly in excess of needs, obtaining sufficient good quality protein is usually only a concern for young children who are not provided with animal proteins.

## Protein Intake

The World Health Organization recommends a daily intake of 0.75 gram of good quality protein per kilogram of body weight for adults of both sexes. Thus, a 70-kg (154-pound) man would need 52.5 grams of protein, and a 55-kg (121-pound) woman would need about 41 grams of protein. This recommendation, based on nitrogen balance studies, assumes an adequate energy intake. Infants, children, and pregnant and lactating women have additional protein needs to support synthesis of new tissue or milk production. Protein requirements of endurance athletes and bodybuilders may be slightly higher than those of sedentary individuals, but this has no practical significance because athletes typically consume much more protein than they need.

Protein consumed in excess of the body's needs is degraded; the nitrogen is excreted as urea, and the remaining keto acids are used for energy, providing 4 kilocalories per gram, or are converted to carbohydrate or fat. During conditions of fasting, starvation, or insufficient dietary intake of protein, lean tissue is broken down to supply amino acids for vital body functions. Persistent protein inadequacy results in suboptimal metabolic function with increased risk of infection and disease.

## Vitamins

Vitamins are organic compounds found in very small amounts in food and required for normal functioning—indeed, for survival. Humans are able to synthesize certain vitamins to some extent. For example, vitamin D is produced when the skin is exposed to sunlight; niacin can be synthesized from the amino acid tryptophan; and vitamin K and biotin are synthesized by bacteria living in the gut. However, in general, humans depend on their diet to supply vitamins. When a vitamin is in short supply or is not able to be utilized properly, a specific deficiency syndrome results. When the deficient vitamin is resupplied before irreversible damage occurs, the signs and symptoms are reversed. The amounts of vitamins in foods and the amounts required on a daily basis are measured in milligrams and micrograms.

Unlike the macronutrients, vitamins do not serve as an energy source for the body or provide raw materials for tissue building. Rather, they assist in energy-yielding reactions and facilitate metabolic and physiologic processes throughout the body. Vitamin A, for example, is required for embryonic development, growth, reproduction, proper immune function, and the integrity of epithelial cells, in addition to its role in vision. The B vitamins function as coenzymes that assist in energy metabolism; folic acid (folate), one of the B vitamins, helps protect against birth defects in the early stages of pregnancy. Vitamin C plays a role in building connective tissue as well as being an antioxidant that helps protect against damage by reactive molecules (free radicals). Now considered to be a hormone, vitamin D is involved in calcium and phosphorus homeostasis and bone metabolism. Vitamin E, another antioxidant, protects against free radical damage in lipid systems, and vitamin K plays a key role in blood clotting. Although vitamins are often discussed individually, many of their functions are interrelated, and a deficiency of one can influence the function of another.

Vitamin nomenclature is somewhat complex, with chemical names gradually replacing the original letter designations created in the era of vitamin discovery during the first half of the 20th century. Nomenclature is further complicated by the recognition that vitamins are parts of families with, in some cases, multiple active forms. Some vitamins are found in foods in precursor forms that must be activated in the body before they can properly fulfill their function. For example, beta($\beta$)-carotene, found in plants, is converted to vitamin A in the body.

The 13 vitamins known to be required by human beings are categorized into two groups according to their solubility. The four fat-soluble vitamins (soluble in nonpolar solvents) are vitamins A, D, E, and K. Although now known to behave as a hormone, the activated form of vitamin D, vitamin D hormone (calcitriol), is still grouped with the vitamins as well. The nine water-soluble vitamins (soluble in polar solvents) are vitamin C and the eight B-complex vitamins: thiamin, riboflavin, niacin, vitamin $B_6$, folic acid, vitamin $B_{12}$, pantothenic acid, and biotin. Choline is a vitamin-like dietary component that is clearly required for normal metabolism but that can be synthesized by the body. Although choline may be necessary in the diet of premature infants and possibly of those with certain medical conditions, it has not been established as essential in the human diet throughout life.

Different vitamins are more or less susceptible to destruction by environmental conditions and chemical agents. For example, thiamin is especially vulnerable to prolonged heating, riboflavin to ultraviolet or fluorescent light, and vitamin C to oxidation (as when a piece of fruit is cut open and the vitamin is exposed to air). In general, water-soluble vitamins are more easily destroyed during cooking than are fat-soluble vitamins.

The solubility of a vitamin influences the way it is absorbed, transported, stored, and excreted by the body as well as where it is found in foods. With the exception of vitamin $B_{12}$, which is supplied by only foods of animal origin, the water-soluble vitamins are synthesized by plants and found in both plant and animal foods. Strict vegetarians (vegans), who eat no foods of animal origin, are therefore at risk of vitamin $B_{12}$ deficiency. Fat-soluble vitamins, on the other hand, are found in association with fats and oils in foods and in the body and typically require protein carriers for transport through the water-filled compartments of the body.

Water-soluble vitamins are not appreciably stored in the body (except for vitamin $B_{12}$) and thus must be consumed regularly in the diet. If taken in excess they are readily excreted in the urine, although there is potential toxicity even with water-soluble vitamins; especially noteworthy in this regard is vitamin $B_6$. Because fat-soluble vitamins are stored in the liver and fatty tissue, they do not necessarily have to be taken in daily, so long as average intakes over time—weeks, months, or even years—meet the body's needs. However, the fact that these vitamins can be stored increases the possibility of toxicity if very large doses are taken. This is particularly of concern with vitamins A and D, which can be toxic if taken in excess. Under certain circumstances, pharmacological ("megadose") levels of some vitamins—many times higher than the amount typically found in food—have accepted medical uses. Niacin, for example, is used to lower blood cholesterol levels; vitamin D is used to treat psoriasis; and pharmacological derivatives of vitamin A are used to treat acne and other skin conditions as well as to diminish skin wrinkling. However, consumption of vitamins or other dietary supplements in amounts significantly in excess of recommended levels is not advised without medical supervision.

Vitamins synthesized in the laboratory are the same molecules as those extracted from food, and they cannot be distinguished by the body. However, various forms of a vitamin are not necessarily equivalent. In the particular case of vitamin E, supplements labeled d-α-tocopherol (or "natural") generally contain more vitamin E activity than those labeled dl-α-tocopherol. Vitamins in food have a distinct advantage over vitamins in supplement form because they come associated with other substances that may be beneficial, and there is also less potential for toxicity. Nutritional supplements cannot substitute for a healthful diet.

## Minerals

Unlike the complex organic compounds (carbohydrates, lipids, proteins, vitamins), minerals are simple inorganic elements—often in the form of salts in the body—that are not themselves metabolized, nor are they a source of energy. Minerals constitute about 4 to 6 percent of body weight—about one-half as calcium and one-quarter as phosphorus (phosphates), the remainder being made up of the other essential minerals that must be derived from the diet. Minerals not only impart hardness to bones and teeth but also function broadly in metabolism—e.g., as electrolytes controlling the movement of water in and out of cells, as components of enzyme systems, and as constituents of many organic molecules.

As nutrients, minerals are traditionally divided into two groups according to the amounts present in and needed by the body. The major minerals (macrominerals)—those required in amounts of 100 milligrams or more per day—are calcium, phosphorus (phosphates), magnesium, sulfur, sodium, chloride, and potassium. The trace elements (microminerals or trace minerals), required in much smaller amounts of about 15 milligrams per day or less, include iron, zinc, copper, manganese, iodine (iodide), selenium, fluoride, molybdenum, chromium, and cobalt (as part of the vitamin $B_{12}$ molecule). Fluoride is considered a beneficial nutrient because of its role in protecting against dental caries, although an essential function in the strict sense has not been established in human nutrition.

The term ultratrace elements is sometimes used to describe minerals that are found in the diet in extremely small quantities (micrograms each day) and are present in human tissue as well; these include arsenic, boron, nickel, silicon, and vanadium. Despite demonstrated roles in experimental animals, the exact function of these and other ultratrace elements (e.g., tin, lithium, aluminum) in human tissues and indeed their importance for human health are uncertain.

Minerals have diverse functions, including muscle contraction, nerve transmission, blood clotting, immunity, the maintenance of blood pressure and growth and development. The major minerals, with the exception of sulfur, typically occur in the body in ionic (charged) form: sodium, potassium, magnesium, and calcium as positive ions (cations) and chloride and phosphates as negative ions (anions). Mineral salts dissolved in body fluids help regulate fluid balance, osmotic pressure, and acid-base balance.

Sulfur, too, has important functions in ionic forms (such as sulfate), but much of the body's sulfur is nonionic, serving as an integral part of certain organic molecules, such as the B vitamins thiamin, biotin, and pantothenic acid and the amino acids methionine, cysteine, and cystine. Other mineral elements that are constituents of organic compounds include iron, which is part of hemoglobin (the oxygen-carrying protein in red blood cells), and iodine, a component of thyroid hormones, which help regulate body metabolism. Additionally, phosphate groups are found in many organic molecules, such as phospholipids in cell membranes, genetic material (DNA and RNA), and the high-energy molecule adenosine triphosphate (ATP).

The levels of different minerals in foods are influenced by growing conditions (e.g., soil and water composition) as well as by how the food is processed. Minerals are not destroyed during food preparation; in fact, a food can be burned completely and the minerals (ash) will remain unchanged. However, minerals can be lost by leaching into cooking water that is subsequently discarded.

Many factors influence mineral absorption and thus availability to the body. In general, minerals are better absorbed from animal foods than from plant foods. The latter contain fibre and other substances that interfere with absorption. Phytic acid, found principally in cereal grains and legumes, can form complexes with some minerals and make them insoluble and thereby indigestible. Only a small percentage of the calcium in spinach is absorbed because spinach also contains large amounts of oxalic acid, which binds calcium. Some minerals, particularly those of a similar size and charge, compete with each other for absorption. For example, iron supplementation may reduce zinc absorption, while excessive intakes of zinc can interfere with copper absorption. On the other hand, the absorption of iron from plants (nonheme iron) is enhanced when vitamin C is simultaneously present in the diet, and calcium absorption is improved by adequate amounts of vitamin D. Another key factor that influences mineral absorption is the physiological need for the mineral at the time.

Unlike many vitamins, which have a broader safety range, minerals can be toxic if taken in doses not far above recommended levels. This is particularly true for the trace elements, such as iron and copper. Accidental ingestion of iron supplements has been a major cause of fatal poisoning in young children.

## Water

Although often overlooked as a nutrient, water ($H_2O$) is actually the most critical nutrient of all. Humans can survive weeks without food but only a matter of days without water.

Water provides the medium in which nutrients and waste products are transported throughout the body and the myriad biochemical reactions of metabolism occur. Water allows for temperature regulation, the maintenance of blood pressure and blood volume, the structure of large molecules, and the rigidity of body tissues. It also acts as a solvent, a lubricant (as in joints), and a protective cushion (as inside the eyes and in spinal fluid and amniotic fluid). The flow of water in and out of cells is precisely controlled by shifting electrolyte concentrations on either side of the cell membrane. Potassium, magnesium, phosphate, and sulfate are primarily intracellular electrolytes; sodium and chloride are major extracellular ones.

Water makes up about 50 to 70 percent of body weight, approximately 60 percent in healthy adults and an even higher percentage in children. Because lean tissue is about three-quarters water, and fatty tissue is only about one-fifth water, body composition—the amount of fat in particular—determines the percentage of body water. In general, men have more lean tissue than women, and therefore a higher percentage of their body weight is water.

Water is consumed not only as water itself and as a constituent of other beverages but also as a major component of many foods, particularly fruits and vegetables, which may contain from 85 to 95 percent water. Water also is manufactured in the body as an end product of metabolism. About 2.5 litres (about 2.6 quarts) of water are turned over daily, with water excretion (primarily in urine, water vapour from lungs, sweat loss from skin, and feces) balancing intake from all sources. Because water requirements vary with climate, level of activity, dietary composition, and other factors, there is no one recommendation for daily water intake. However, adults typically need at least 2 litres (8 cups) of water a day, from all sources. Thirst is not reliable as a register for dehydration, which typically occurs before the body is prompted to replace fluid. Therefore, water intake is advised throughout the day, especially with increased sweat loss in hot climates or during vigorous physical activity, during illness, or in a dehydrating situation such as an airplane flight.

## Food Groups

The following nine food groups reflect foods with generally similar nutritional characteristics: (1) cereals, (2) starchy roots, (3) legumes, (4) vegetables and fruits, (5) sugars, preserves, and syrups, (6) meat, fish, and eggs, (7) milk and milk products, (8) fats and oils, and (9) beverages.

## Cereals

The cereals are all grasses that have been bred over millennia to bear large seeds (i.e., grain). The most important cereals for human consumption are rice, wheat, and corn (maize). Others include barley, oats, and millet. The carbohydrate-rich cereals compare favourably with the protein-rich foods in energy value; in addition, the cost of production (per calorie) of cereals is less than that of almost all other foods and they can be stored dry for many years. Therefore, most of the world's diets are arranged to meet main calorie requirements from the cheaper carbohydrate foods. The major component of all grains is starch. Cereals contain little fat, with oats having an exceptional 9 percent. The amount of protein in cereals ranges from 6 to 16 percent but does not have as high a nutritive value as that of many animal foods because of the low lysine content.

Controversy exists as to the relative merits of white bread and bread made from whole wheat flour. White flour consists of about 72 percent of the grain but contains little of the germ (embryo) and of the outer coverings (bran). Since the B vitamins are concentrated mainly in the scutellum (covering of the germ), and to a lesser extent in the bran, the vitamin B content of white flour, unless artificially enriched, is less than that of brown flour. Dietary fibre is located mostly in the bran, so that white flour contains only about one-third of that in whole wheat flour. White flour is compulsorily enriched with synthetic vitamins in a number of countries, including the United States and the United Kingdom, so that the vitamin content is similar to that of the darker flours. White flour, of course, still lacks fibre and any yet unidentified beneficial factors that may be present in the outer layers of the wheat.

B vitamins are also lost when brown rice is polished to yield white rice. People living on white rice and little else are at risk for developing the disease beriberi, which is caused by a deficiency of thiamin (vitamin $B_1$). Beriberi was formerly common in poor Asian communities in which a large proportion of the diet consisted of polished rice. The disease has almost completely disappeared from Asia with the advent of greater availability of other foods and, in some areas, fortification of the rice with thiamin.

Yellow corn differs from other cereals in that it contains carotenoids with vitamin A activity. (Another exception is a genetically modified so-called golden rice, which contains carotene, the precursor for vitamin A). Corn is also lower in the amino acid tryptophan than other cereals. The niacin in corn is in a bound form that cannot be digested or absorbed by humans unless pretreated with lime (calcium hydroxide) or unless immature grains are eaten at the so-called milky stage (usually as sweet corn). Niacin is also formed in the body as a metabolite of the amino acid tryptophan, but this alternative source is not available when the tryptophan content is too low.

## Starchy Roots

Starchy roots consumed in large quantities include potatoes, sweet potatoes, yams, taro, and cassava. Their nutritive value in general resembles that of cereals. The potato, however, provides some protein (2 percent) and also contains vitamin C. The yellow-fleshed varieties of sweet potato contain the pigment beta-carotene, convertible in the body into vitamin A. Cassava is extremely low in protein, and most varieties contain cyanide-forming compounds that make them toxic unless processed correctly.

## Legumes

Beans and peas are the seeds of leguminous crops that are able to utilize atmospheric nitrogen via parasitic microorganisms attached to their roots. Legumes contain at least 20 percent protein, and they are a good source of most of the B vitamins and of iron. Like cereals, most legumes are low in fat; an important exception is the soybean (17 percent), a major commercial source of edible oil. Tofu, or bean curd, is made from soybeans and is an important source of protein in China, Japan, Korea, and Southeast Asia. Peanuts (groundnuts) are also the seeds of a leguminous plant, although they ripen underground; much of the crop is processed for its oil.

## Vegetables and Fruits

Vegetables and fruits have similar nutritive properties. Because 70 percent or more of their weight is water, they provide comparatively little energy or protein, but many contain vitamin C and carotene. However, cooked vegetables are an uncertain source of vitamin C, as this vitamin is easily destroyed by heat. The dark-green leafy vegetables are particularly good sources of vitamin A activity. Vegetables also provide calcium and iron but often in a form that is poorly absorbed. The more typical fruits, such as apples, oranges, and berries, are rich in sugar. Bananas are a good source of potassium. Vegetables and fruits also contain fibre, which adds bulk to the intestinal content and is useful in preventing constipation.

Botanically, nuts are actually a kind of fruit, but they are quite different in character with their hard shell and high fat content. The coconut, for example, contains some 60 percent fat when dried. Olives are another fruit rich in fat and are traditionally grown for their oil.

## Sugars, Preserves and Syrups

One characteristic of diets of affluent societies is their high content of sugar. This is due in part to sugar added at the table or as an ingredient in candy, preserves, and sweetened colas or other beverages. There are also naturally occurring sugars in foods (lactose in milk and fructose, glucose, and sucrose in fruits and some vegetables). Sugar, however, contains no protein, minerals, or vitamins and thus has been called the source of "empty calories."

Because sugar adsorbs water and prevents the growth of microorganisms, it is an excellent preservative. Making jam or marmalade is a way of preserving fruit, but most of the vitamin C is destroyed, and the products contain up to 70 percent sugar. Honey and natural syrups (e.g., maple syrup) are composed of more than 75 percent sugar.

## Meat, Fish and Eggs

Generally meats consist of about 20 percent protein, 20 percent fat, and 60 percent water. The amount of fat present in a particular portion of meat varies greatly, not only with the kind of meat but also with the quality; has the "energy value" varied in direct proportion with the fat content. Meat is valuable for its protein, which is of high biological value. Pork is an excellent source of thiamin. Meat is also a good source of niacin, vitamin $B_{12}$, vitamin $B_6$, and the mineral nutrients iron, zinc, phosphorus, potassium, and magnesium. Liver is the storage organ for, and is very rich in, vitamin A, riboflavin, and folic acid. In many cultures the organs (offal) of animals—including the kidneys, the heart, the tongue, and the liver—are considered delicacies. Liver is a particularly rich source of many vitamins.

The muscular tissue of fishes consists of 13 to 20 percent protein, fat ranging from less than 1 to more than 20 percent, and 60 to 82 percent water that varies inversely with fat content. Many species of fish, such as cod and haddock, concentrate fat in the liver and as a result have extremely lean muscles. The tissues of other fish, such as salmon and herring, may contain 15 percent fat or more. However, fish oil, unlike the fat in land animals, is rich in essential long-chain fatty acids, particularly eicosapentaenoic acid.

The egg has a deservedly high reputation as a food. Its white contains protein, and its yolk is rich in both protein and vitamin A. An egg also provides calcium and iron. Egg yolk, however, has a high cholesterol content.

## Milk and Milk Products

The milk of each species of animal is a complete food for its young. Moreover, one pint of cow's milk contributes about 90 percent of the calcium, 30 to 40 percent of the riboflavin, 25 to 30 percent of the protein, 10 to 20 percent of the calories and vitamins A and B, and up to 10 percent of the iron and vitamin D needed by a human adult.

Human breast milk is the perfect food for infants, provided it comes from a healthy, well-nourished mother and the infant is full-term. Breast milk contains important antibodies, white blood cells, and nutrients. In communities where hygiene is poor, breast-fed babies have fewer infections than formula-fed babies. In the past, infants who could not be breast-fed were given cow's milk that was partially "humanized" with the addition of water and a small amount of sugar or wheat flour. However, this was far from an ideal substitute for breast milk, being lower in iron and containing undenatured proteins that could produce allergic reactions with bleeding into the gut and, in some cases, eczema.

Lactose, the characteristic sugar of milk, is a disaccharide made of the monosaccharides glucose and galactose. Some adults can break down the lactose of large quantities of milk into galactose and glucose, but others have an inherited lactose intolerance as a result of the lactase enzyme no longer being secreted into the gut after the age of weaning. As a result, unabsorbed lactose is fermented by bacteria and produces bloating and gas. People who have little lactase in their bodies can still consume large amounts of milk if it has been allowed to go sour, if lactobacilli have split most of the lactose into lactic acid (as in yogurt), or if the lactose has been treated with commercially available lactase. People originating in northern Europe usually retain full intestinal lactase activity into adult life.

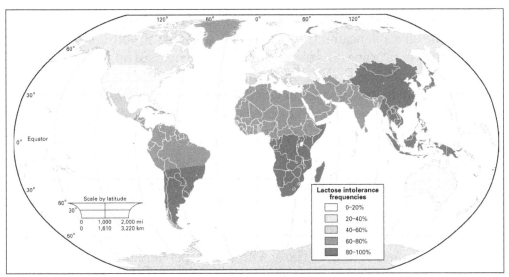

Lactose intolerance, global distribution. Global distribution of lactose intolerance in humans.

Most commercially available milk has been pasteurized with heat to kill bovine tuberculosis organisms and other possible pathogens. The most widely used method for pasteurizing milk is the high-temperature, short-time (HTST) sterilization treatment. If products are to be stored under refrigeration, or even at room temperature, for long periods of time, they may be processed by ultrahigh temperature (UHT) pasteurization. Another method of preserving milk without refrigeration involves the removal of water to form condensed milk, which can be exposed to air for several days without deterioration. Milk, either whole or defatted, can also be dried to a powder. In some countries, such as the United States, milk is homogenized so that fat particles are broken up and evenly distributed throughout the product.

Cow's milk is good food for human adults, but the cream (i.e., the fat) contains 52 percent saturated fatty acids as compared with only 3 percent polyunsaturated fat. This fat is either drunk with the milk or eaten in butter or cream. Because milk fat is regarded as undesirable by people who want to reduce their energy intake or cholesterol level, the dairy industry has developed low-fat cow's milk (with 2 percent fat instead of the almost 4 percent of whole milk), very low-fat skim milk, and skim milk with extra nonfat milk solids (lactose, protein, and calcium) that give more body to the milk. Buttermilk, originally the watery residue of butter making, is now made from either low-fat or skim milk that has been inoculated with nonpathogenic bacteria.

Cheese making is an ancient art formerly used on farms to convert surplus milk into a food that could be stored without refrigeration. Rennet, an enzyme found in a calf's stomach, is added to milk, causing the milk protein casein to coagulate into a semisolid substance called curd, thus trapping most of the fat. The remaining watery liquid (whey) is then drained, and the curd is salted, inoculated with nonpathogenic organisms, and allowed to dry and mature. Cheese is rich in protein and calcium and is a good source of vitamin A and riboflavin. Most cheeses, however, contain about 25 to 30 percent fat (constituting about 70 percent of the calories of the cheese), which is mostly saturated, and they are usually high in sodium.

## Fats and Oils

The animal fats used by humans are butter, suet (beef fat), lard (pork fat), and fish oils. Important vegetable oils include olive oil, peanut (groundnut) oil, coconut oil, cottonseed oil, sunflower seed oil, soybean oil, safflower oil, rape oil, sesame (gingelly) oil, mustard oil, red palm oil, and corn oil. Fats and oils provide more calories per gram than any other food, but they contain no protein and few micronutrients. Only butter and the previously mentioned fish-liver oils contain any vitamin A or D, though red palm oil does contain carotene, which is converted to vitamin A in the body. Vitamins A and D are added to margarines. All natural fats and oils contain variable amounts of vitamin E, the fat-soluble vitamin antioxidant.

The predominant substances in fats and oils are triglycerides, chemical compounds containing any three fatty acids combined with a molecule of glycerol. When no double bonds are present, a fatty acid is said to be saturated; with the presence of one or more double bonds, a fatty acid is said to be unsaturated. Fats with a high percentage of saturated fatty acids, e.g., butter and lard, tend to be solid at room temperature. Those with a high percentage of unsaturated fatty acids are usually liquid oils, e.g., sunflower, safflower, and corn oils. The process of hydrogenation is used by the food industry to convert unsaturated oils to saturated solid fats, which are more resistant to rancidity. However, hydrogenation also causes the formation of trans-fatty acids. These appear to have some of the same undesirable effects on blood cholesterol as saturated fatty acids.

A small group of fatty acids is essential in the diet. They occur in body structures, especially the different membranes inside and around cells, and cannot be synthesized in the body from other fats. Linoleic acid is the most important of these fatty acids because it is convertible to other essential fatty acids. Linoleic acid has two double bonds and is a polyunsaturated fatty acid. As well as being an essential fatty acid, it tends to lower the cholesterol level in the blood. Linoleic acid occurs in moderate to high proportions in many of the seed oils, e.g., corn, sunflower, cottonseed, and safflower oils. Some margarine (polyunsaturated margarines) use a blend of oils selected to provide moderately high linoleic acid content.

## Beverages

Although most adults drink one to two litres (about one to two quarts) of water a day, much of this is in the form of liquids such as coffee, tea, fruit juices, and soft drinks. In general, these are appreciated more for their taste or for their effects than for their nutritive value. Fruit juices are useful for their vitamin C content and are good sources of potassium; however, they tend to be very high in sugar. Coffee and tea by themselves are of little nutritive value; coffee contains some niacin, and tea contains fluoride and manganese. These beverages also contain natural caffeine, which has a stimulating effect. Caffeine is added to colas, and so-called diet soft drinks contain small quantities of artificial sweeteners in place of sugars so that their overall calorie value is reduced.

Since ethyl alcohol (ethanol) has an energy value of 7 kilocalories per gram, very significant amounts of energy can be obtained from alcoholic drinks. Beer contains 2 to 6 percent alcohol, wines 10 to 13 percent, and most spirits up to 40 percent. Fermented drinks also include significant amounts of residual sugars, and champagne and dessert wines may have sugar added to them. With one or two exceptions, alcoholic beverages contain no nutrients and are only a source of "empty calories." The only vitamin present in significant amounts in beer is riboflavin. Wines are devoid of vitamins but sometimes contain large amounts of iron, probably acquired from iron vessels used in their preparation. Heavy alcohol consumption is known to lead to a greater risk of malnutrition, in part because it can damage the absorptive power of the gut and also because heavy drinkers commonly neglect to follow a normal pattern of meals. On the other hand, evidence from a number of studies shows that persons consuming one to two drinks per day are healthier than are those who abstain from drinking alcohol. This might be due in part to substances in red wine, such as flavonoids and tannins, which may protect against heart disease.

Table: Comparison of energy, carbohydrates, and alcohol in some common beverages.

| Beverage | Typical volume (fl oz) | Energy (kcal) | Carbohydrates (g) | Alcohol (g) |
|---|---|---|---|---|
| Beer | 12 | 100–150 | 3–15 | 12 |
| Club soda | 12 | 0 | 0 | 0 |
| Cocktails | 3.5 | 120–180 | 4–8 | 18–24 |
| Colas | 12 | 150 | 40 | 0 |
| Colas, diet | 12 | 2 | 0 | 0 |
| Ginger ale | 12 | 120 | 30 | 0 |
| Milk, whole | 8 | 150 | 11 | 0 |
| Milk, skim | 8 | 85 | 12 | 0 |
| Spirits | 1.5 | 100–120 | 0 | 15–17 |
| Wine, dessert | 3.5 | 130–160 | 4–12 | 11 |
| Wine, dry | 3.5 | 70–80 | 3–4 | 11 |

## Dietary and Nutrient Recommendations

Notions of what constitutes a healthful diet vary with geography and custom as well as with changing times and an evolving understanding of nutrition. In the past, people had to live almost entirely on food that was locally produced. With industrialization and globalization, however, food can now be transported over long distances. Researchers must be careful in making generalizations about a national diet from a relatively small sample of the population; the poor cannot afford to eat the same diet as the rich, and many countries have large immigrant groups with their own distinctive food patterns. Even within a culture, some people abstain on moral or religious grounds from eating certain foods. In general, persons living in more affluent countries eat more meat and other animal products. By comparison, the diets of those living in poorer, agricultural countries rely primarily on cereals in the form of wheat flour, white rice, or corn, with animal products providing less than 10 percent of energy. Another difference between cultures is the extent to which dairy products are consumed. The Chinese, for example, obtain about 2 percent of their energy from dairy products. In contrast, in Pakistan dairy products contribute almost 10 percent of energy. Among Western diets, the lowest in saturated fat is the so-called Mediterranean diet. In the 1950s it was found that Europeans living in rural areas near the Mediterranean Sea had a greater life expectancy than those living elsewhere in Europe, despite poor medical services and a lower standard of living. The traditional diet of Mediterranean peoples is low in animal products; instead, olive oil is a major source of monounsaturated fat. Also, tomatoes and green leafy vegetables, which are regularly consumed in large quantities in the region, contain a variety of antioxidant compounds that are thought to be healthful.

## Dietary Guidelines

Following the publication of dietary goals for the Nordic countries in 1968 and for the United States in 1977, dietary goals and guidelines have been set forth by a number of countries and revised periodically as a way of translating scientific recommendations into simple and practical dietary suggestions. These authoritative statements—some published by scientific bodies and some by government agencies—aim to promote long-term health and to prevent or reduce the chances of developing chronic and degenerative diseases. Although the guidelines of different countries may vary in important ways, most recent dietary recommendations include variations on the following fundamental themes: eat a variety of foods; perform regular physical activity and maintain a healthy weight; limit consumption of saturated fat, trans fat, sugar, salt (more specifically, sodium), and alcohol; and emphasize vegetables, fruits, and whole grains.

## Food Guide Pyramids and other Aids

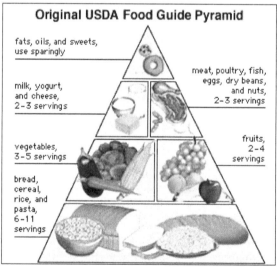

The original USDA Food Guide Pyramid recommended a liberal daily intake
of grain products (represented by the wide base of the pyramid) and a sparing
intake of fats, oils, and sugary foods (represented by the tip of the structure).

Different formats for dietary goals and guidelines have been developed over the years as educational tools, grouping foods of similar nutrient content together to help facilitate the selection of a balanced diet. In the United States, the four food-group plan of the 1950s—which suggested a milk group, a meat group, a fruit and vegetable group, and a breads and cereals group as a basic diet—was replaced in 1992 by the five major food groups of the Food Guide Pyramid. This innovative visual display was introduced by the United States Department of Agriculture (USDA) as a tool for helping the public cultivate a daily pattern of wise food choices, ranging from liberal consumption of grain products, as represented in the broad base of the pyramid, to sparing use of fats, oils, and sugary foods, as represented in the apex. Subsequently, similar devices were developed for particular cultural and ethnic food patterns such as Asian, Latin American, Mediterranean, and even vegetarian diets—all emphasizing grains, vegetables, and fruits. While an adaptation of the 1992 USDA pyramid was used by Mexico, Chile, the Philippines, and Panama, a rainbow was used by Canada, a square by Zimbabwe, plates by Australia and the United Kingdom, a bean pot by Guatemala, the number 6 by Japan, and a pagoda by South Korea and China.

In the early 21st century, many countries altered the pictorial representation of their food guides. For example, in 2005 Japan introduced a spinning-top food guide that essentially was an inverted version of the U.S. pyramid graphic. That same year, the USDA released new dietary guidelines and redesigned its original Food Guide Pyramid, which was known as MyPyramid and featured colorful vertical stripes of varying widths to reflect the relative proportions of different food groups. Similar to Japan's spinning-top graphic, which depicted a figure running on the top's upper level, the MyPyramid graphic used a figure climbing steps to illustrate the importance of daily exercise. Unlike the original Food Guide Pyramid, the abstract geometry of MyPyramid did not offer specific dietary guidance at a glance; rather, individuals were directed to an interactive Web site for customized eating plans based on their age, sex, and activity level.

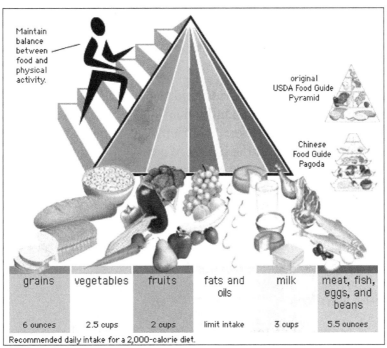

Food Guide Pyramid: MyPyramid, introduced by the U.S. Department of Agriculture in 2005, represented the major food groups in vertical bands. It was replaced in 2011 by a revised food guide graphic known as MyPlate.

In 2011 the USDA abandoned MyPyramid and introduced MyPlate, which divided the four basic food groups (fruits, grains, protein, and vegetables) into sections on a plate, with the size of each section representing the relative dietary proportions of each food group. A small circle shown at the edge of the plate was used to illustrate the dietary inclusion and proportion of dairy products. Unlike MyPyramid, MyPlate did not include an exercise component, nor did it include a section for fats and oils. The two were similar, however, in that the guidance they offered was nonspecific and was supported by a website.

## Adapting Guidelines to Culture

Dietary guidelines have been largely the province of more affluent countries, where correcting imbalances due to overconsumption and inappropriate food choices has been key. Not until 1989 were proposals for dietary guidelines published from the perspective of low-income countries, such as India, where the primary nutrition problems stemmed from the lack of opportunity to acquire or consume needed food. But even in such countries, there was a growing risk of obesity and chronic disease among the small but increasing number of affluent people who had adopted some of the dietary habits of the industrialized world. For example, the Chinese Dietary Guidelines, published by the Chinese Nutrition Society in 1997, made recommendations for that part of the population dealing with nutritional diseases such as those resulting from iodine and vitamin A deficiencies, for people in some remote areas where there was a lack of food, as well as for the urban population coping with changing lifestyle, dietary excess, and increasing rates of chronic disease. The Food Guide Pagoda, a graphic display intended to help Chinese consumers put the dietary recommendations into practice, rested on the traditional cereal-based Chinese diet. Those who could not tolerate fresh milk were encouraged to consume yogurt or other dairy products as a source of calcium. Unlike dietary recommendations in Western countries, the pagoda did not include sugar, as sugar consumption by the Chinese was quite low; however, children and adolescents in particular were cautioned to limit sugar intake because of the risk of dental caries.

## Nutrient Recommendations

The relatively simple dietary guidelines provide guidance for meal planning. Standards for evaluating the adequacy of specific nutrients in an individual diet or the diet of a population require more detailed and quantitative recommendations. Nutrient recommendations are usually determined by scientific bodies within a country at the behest of government agencies. The World Health Organization and other agencies of the United Nations have also issued reports on nutrients and food components. The Recommended Dietary Allowances (RDAs), first published by the U.S. National Academy of Sciences in 1941 and revised every few years until 1989, established dietary standards for evaluating nutritional intakes of populations and for planning food supplies. The RDAs reflected the best scientific judgment of the time in setting amounts of different nutrients adequate to meet the nutritional needs of most healthy people.

## Dietary Reference Intakes

During the 1990s a paradigm shift took place as scientists from the United States and Canada joined forces in an ambitious multiyear project to reframe dietary standards for the two countries. In the revised approach, known as the Dietary Reference Intakes (DRIs), classic indicators of deficiency, such as scurvy and beriberi, were considered an insufficient basis for recommendations. Where warranted by a sufficient research base, the guidelines rely on indicators with broader significance, those that might reflect a decreased risk of chronic diseases such as osteoporosis, heart disease, hypertension, or cancer. DRIs are intended to help individuals plan a healthful diet as well as avoid consuming too much of a nutrient. The comprehensive approach of the DRIs has served as a model for other countries. A DRI report was published in 1997, and subsequent updates were published for specific nutrients and for some food components such as flavonoids that are not considered nutrients but have an impact on health.

The collective term Dietary Reference Intakes encompasses four categories of reference values. The Estimated Average Requirement (EAR) is the intake level for a nutrient at which the needs of 50 percent of the population will be met. Because the needs of the other half of the population will not be met by this amount, the EAR is increased by about 20 percent to arrive at the RDA. The RDA is the average daily dietary intake level sufficient to meet the nutrient requirement of nearly all (97 to 98 percent) healthy persons in a particular life stage. When the EAR, and thus the RDA, cannot be set due to insufficient scientific evidence, another parameter, the Adequate Intake (AI), is given, based on estimates of intake levels of healthy populations. Lastly, the Tolerable Upper Intake Level (UL) is the highest level of a daily nutrient intake that will most likely present no risk of adverse health effects in almost all individuals in the general population.

Table: Tolerable upper intake level (UL) for selected nutrients for adults.

| Nutrient | Ul per day |
|---|---|
| Calcium | 2,500 milligrams |
| Copper | 10 milligrams |
| Fluoride | 10 milligrams |
| Folic acid | 1,000 micrograms |
| Iodine | 1,100 micrograms |
| Iron | 45 milligrams |
| Magnesium | 350 milligrams |
| Manganese | 11 milligrams |
| Niacin | 35 milligrams |
| Phosphorus | 4 grams |
| Selenium | 400 micrograms |
| Vitamin A | 3,000 micrograms (10,000 IU) |
| Vitamin B$_6$ | 100 milligrams |
| Vitamin C | 2,000 milligrams |
| Vitamin D | 50 micrograms (2,000 IU) |
| Vitamin E | 1,000 milligrams |
| Zinc | 40 milligrams |

Nutrition information is commonly displayed on food labels, but this information is generally simplified to avoid confusion. Because only one nutrient reference value is listed, and because sex and age categories usually are not taken into consideration, the amount chosen is generally the highest RDA value. In the United States, for example, the Daily Values, determined by the Food and Drug Administration, are generally based on RDA values published in 1968. The different food components are listed on the food label as a percentage of their Daily Values.

Confidence that a desirable level of intake is reasonable for a particular group of people can be bolstered by multiple lines of evidence pointing in the same direction, an understanding of the function of the nutrient and how it is handled by the body, and a comprehensive theoretical model with strong statistical underpinnings. Of critical importance in estimating nutrient requirements is explicitly defining the criterion that the specified level of intake is intended to satisfy. Approaches that use different definitions of adequacy are not comparable. For example, it is one thing to prevent clinical impairment of bodily function (basal requirement), which does not necessarily require any reserves of the nutrient, but it is another to consider an amount that will provide desirable reserves (normative requirement) in the body. Yet another approach attempts to evaluate a nutrient intake conducive to optimal health, even if an amount is required beyond that normally obtainable in food—possibly necessitating the use of supplements. Furthermore, determining upper levels of safe intake requires evidence of a different sort. These issues are extremely complex, and the scientists who collaborate to set nutrient recommendations face exceptional challenges in their attempts to reach consensus.

## Nutrition Throughout the Life Cycle

Nutritional needs and concerns vary during different stages of life.

## Pregnancy and Lactation

A woman's nutritional status before and during pregnancy affects not only her own health but also the health and development of her baby. If a woman is underweight before becoming pregnant or fails to gain sufficient weight during pregnancy, her chance of having a premature or low-birth-weight infant is increased. Overweight women, on the other hand, have a high risk of complications during pregnancy, such as high blood pressure (hypertension) and gestational diabetes, and of having a poorly developed infant or one with birth defects. Weight loss during pregnancy is never recommended. Recommended weight gain during pregnancy is 11.5 to 16 kg (25 to 35 pounds) for a woman of normal weight—slightly more for an underweight woman and slightly less for an overweight woman.

At critical periods in the development of specific organs and tissues, there is increased vulnerability to nutrient deficiencies, nutrient excesses, or toxins. For example, excess vitamin A taken early in pregnancy can cause brain malformations in the fetus. One important medical advance of the late 20th century was the recognition that a generous intake of folic acid (also called folate or folacin) in early pregnancy reduces the risk of birth defects, specifically neural tube defects such as spina bifida and anencephaly (partial or complete absence of the brain), which involve spinal cord damage and varying degrees of paralysis, if not death. For this reason, supplementation with 400 micrograms (0.4 milligram) of folic acid is recommended for all women who have a chance of becoming pregnant. Good food sources of folic acid include green leafy vegetables, citrus fruit and juice, beans and other legumes, whole grains, fortified breakfast cereals, and liver.

Overall nutritional requirements increase with pregnancy. In the second and third trimesters, pregnant women need additional food energy—about 300 kilocalories above nonpregnant needs. Most additional nutrient needs can be met by selecting food wisely, but an iron supplement (30 milligrams per day) is usually recommended during the second and third trimesters, in addition to a folic acid supplement throughout pregnancy. Other key nutrients of particular concern are protein, vitamin D, calcium, and zinc.

Heavy alcohol consumption or "binge drinking" during pregnancy can cause fetal alcohol syndrome, a condition with irreversible mental and physical retardation. Even lighter social drinking during pregnancy may result in milder damage—growth retardation, behavioral or learning abnormalities, or motor impairments—sometimes described as fetal alcohol effects. Until a completely safe level of intake can be determined, pregnant women are advised not to drink at all, especially during the first trimester. Caffeine consumption is usually limited as a precautionary measure, and cigarette smoking is not advised under any circumstances. Limiting intake of certain fish, such as swordfish and shark, which may be contaminated with methylmercury, is also recommended.

An extra 500 kilocalories of food per day is needed to meet the energy demands of lactation. Because pregnancy depletes maternal iron stores, iron supplementation during lactation may be advised. Breast-fed infants may be sensitive to the constituents and flavors of foods and beverages consumed by the mother. In general, lactating women are advised to consume little, if any, alcohol.

## Infancy, Childhood and Adolescence

Breast-fed infants, in general, have fewer infections and a reduced chance of developing allergies and food intolerances. For these and other reasons, breast-feeding is strongly recommended for at least the first four to six months of life. However, if a woman is unable to breast-feed or chooses not to, infant formulas (altered forms of cow's milk) can provide safe and adequate nourishment for an infant. Goat's milk, evaporated milk, and sweetened condensed milk are inappropriate for infants. Soy formulas and hydrolyzed protein formulas can be used if a milk allergy is suspected. In developing countries with poor sanitation, over-diluted formulas or those prepared with contaminated water can cause malnutrition and infection, resulting in diarrhea, dehydration, and even death. Breast-fed infants may need supplements of iron and vitamin D during the first six months of life and fluoride after six months. A vitamin $B_{12}$ supplement is advised for breast-fed infants whose mothers are strict vegetarians (vegans).

Solid foods, starting with iron-fortified infant cereals, can be introduced between four and six months to meet nutrient needs that breast milk or infant formulas can no longer supply alone. Other foods can be introduced gradually, one every few days. Infants should not be given honey (which may contain bacteria that can cause botulism), foods that are too salty or sweet, foods that may cause choking, or large amounts of fruit juice.

Starting at one year of age, whole cow's milk can be an excellent source of nutrients for children. However, because cow's milk is associated with gastrointestinal blood loss, iron deficiency, and an allergic response in some young infants, some medical societies do not recommend giving unmodified whole cow's milk to children less than one year old. Low-fat or nonfat milk is inappropriate for children less than two years of age.

The rapid growth rate of infancy slows down in early childhood. During childhood—but not before the age of two—a gradual transition to lower-fat foods is recommended, along with regular exercise. Establishing healthful practices in childhood will reduce the risk of childhood obesity as well as obesity in adulthood and related chronic diseases (e.g., heart disease, diabetes, and high blood pressure).

Vegetarian children can be well nourished but care is needed for them to receive sufficient energy (calories), good-quality protein, vitamins $B_{12}$ and D, and the minerals iron, zinc, and calcium. It is difficult for children who do not drink milk to obtain enough calcium from their food, and supplements may be required. Because of possible toxicity, iron supplements should be taken only under medical supervision.

A small percentage of school-age children who have difficulty sitting still and paying attention are diagnosed with attention-deficit/ hyperactivity disorder (ADHD). Studies have found no convincing evidence that ADHD is caused by sugar or food additives in the diet or that symptoms can be alleviated by eliminating these substances.

Because of unusual eating practices, skipped meals, and concerns about body image, many teenagers, especially girls, have a less than optimal diet. Teenage girls, in particular, need to take special care to obtain adequate amounts of calcium so that bones can be properly mineralized. Iron-deficiency anemia is a concern not only for teenage girls, who lose iron periodically in menstrual blood, but also for teenage boys.

## Adulthood

No matter which nutritional and health practices are followed, the body continues to age, and there appears to be a strong genetic component to life expectancy. Nevertheless, healthful dietary practices and habits such as limited alcohol use, avoidance of tobacco products, and regular physical activity can help reduce the chance of premature death and increase the chance of vitality in the older years. For the most part, a diet that is beneficial for adults in general is also beneficial for people as they age, taking into account possible changes in energy needs.

In elderly people, common problems that contribute to inadequate nutrition are tooth loss, decreased sense of taste and smell, and a sense of isolation—all of which result in decreased food intake and weight loss. The elderly may have gastrointestinal ailments, such as poor absorption of vitamin $B_{12}$, and digestion difficulties, such as constipation. Inadequate fluid intake may lead to dehydration. Nutritional deficiency may further compromise declining immune function. Prescription and over-the-counter drugs may interact with nutrients and exacerbate the nutritional deficits of the elderly. In addition, decreasing physical activity, loss of muscle tissue, and increasing body fat are associated with type 2 diabetes, hypertension, and risk of cardiovascular disease and other diseases. Older people, especially those with reduced sun exposure or low intakes of fatty fish or vitamin D-fortified food, may need supplemental vitamin D to help preserve bone mass. Adequate calcium intake and weight-bearing exercise are also important, but these measures cannot completely stop the decline in bone density with age that makes both men and women vulnerable to bone fractures (due to osteoporosis), which could leave them bedridden and could even be life-threatening. Treatment with various bone-conserving drugs has been found to be effective in slowing bone loss. Staying physically fit as one ages can improve strength and balance, thereby preventing falls, contributing to overall health, and reducing the impact of aging.

There is evidence that intake of the antioxidants vitamin C, vitamin E, and beta-carotene as well as the mineral zinc may slow the progression of age-related macular degeneration, a leading cause of blindness in people older than 65 years. Two carotenoids, lutein and zeaxanthin, also are being studied for their possible role in protecting against age-related vision loss. Research suggests that the dietary supplement glucosamine, a substance that occurs naturally in the body and contributes to cartilage formation, may be useful in lessening the pain and disability of osteoarthritis. Aerobic exercise and strength training, as well as losing excess weight, also may provide some relief from arthritis pain.

Elevated blood levels of the amino acid homocysteine have been associated with an increased risk of cardiovascular disease and with Alzheimer disease, the most common form of dementia; certain B vitamins, particularly folic acid, may be effective in lowering homocysteine levels. High concentrations of aluminum in the brains of persons with Alzheimer disease are most likely a result of the disease and not a cause, as correspondingly high levels of aluminum are not found in blood and hair. There is ongoing research into the possible value of dietary supplements for the normal memory problems that beset healthy older people.

Eating a healthful diet, obtaining sufficient sleep, avoiding smoking, keeping physically fit, and maintaining an active mind are among the practices that may increase not only life expectancy but also the chance of a full and productive life in one's later years. The so-called free-radical theory of aging—the notion that aging is accelerated by highly reactive substances that damage cellular components, and that intake of various antioxidants can repair free-radical damage and thereby slow aging—has generated much interest and is a promising area of research, but it has not been scientifically established. On the contrary, the life spans of various mammalian species have not been extended significantly by antioxidant therapy. Ongoing studies are investigating whether the consumption of 30 percent fewer calories (undernutrition, not malnutrition) slows aging and age-related disease and extends life spans in nonhuman primates. There is no evidence that severe energy restriction would extend the human life span beyond its current maximum of 115 to 120 years.

## Malnutrition

Malnutrition results from a poor diet or a lack of food. It happens when the intake of nutrients or energy is too high, too low, or poorly balanced. Undernutrition can lead to delayed growth or wasting, while a diet that provides too much food, but not necessarily balanced, leads to obesity.

In many parts of the world, undernutrition results from a lack of food. In some cases, however, undernourishment may stem from a health condition, such as an eating disorder or a chronic illness that prevents the person from absorbing nutrients.

According to the World Health Organization (WHO), malnutrition is the gravest single threat to global public health. Globally, it contributes to 45 percent of deaths of children aged under 5 years. Malnutrition involves a dietary deficiency. People may eat too much of the wrong type of food and have malnutrition, when a person lacks nutrients because they do not consume enough food.

Poor diet may lead to a lack of vitamins, minerals, and other essential substances. Too little protein can lead to kwashiorkor, symptoms of which include a distended abdomen. A lack of vitamin C can result in scurvy. Scurvy is rare in industrialized nations, but it can affect older people, those who consume excessive quantities of alcohol, and people who do not eat fresh fruits and vegetables. Some infants and children who follow a limited diet for any reason may be prone to scurvy.

According to the World Health Organization (WHO), 462 million people worldwide are malnourished, and stunted development due to poor diet affects 159 million children globally. Malnutrition during childhood can lead not only to long-term health problems but also to educational challenges and limited work opportunities in the future. Malnourished children often have smaller babies when they grow up. It can also slow recovery from wounds and illnesses, and it can complicate diseases such as measles, pneumonia, malaria, and diarrhea. It can leave the body more susceptible to disease.

## Symptoms

Signs and symptoms of undernutrition include:

- Lack of appetite or interest in food or drink.

- Tiredness and irritability.

- Inability to concentrate.

- Always feeling cold.

- Loss of fat, muscle mass and body tissue.

- Higher risk of getting sick and taking longer to heal.

- Longer healing time for wounds.

- Higher risk of complications after surgery.

- Depression.

- Reduced sex drive and problems with fertility.

In more severe cases:

- Breathing becomes difficult.

- Skin may become thin, dry, inelastic, pale, and cold.

- The cheeks appear hollow and the eyes sunken, as fat disappears from the face.

- Hair becomes dry and sparse, falling out easily.

Eventually, there may be respiratory failure and heart failure, and the person may become unresponsive. Total starvation can be fatal within 8 to 12 weeks.

Children may show a lack of growth, and they may be tired and irritable. Behavioral and intellectual development may be slow, possibly resulting in learning difficulties. Even with treatment, there can be long-term effects on mental function, and digestive problems may persist. In some cases, these may be lifelong.

Adults with severe undernourishment that started during adulthood usually make a full recovery with treatment.

## Causes

Malnutrition can result from various environmental and medical conditions:

- Low intake of food: This may be caused by symptoms of an illness, for example, dysphagia, when it is difficult to swallow. Badly fitting dentures may contribute.

- Mental health problems: Conditions such as depression, dementia, schizophrenia, anorexia nervosa, and bulimia can lead to malnutrition.

- Social and mobility problems: Some people cannot leave the house to buy food or find it physically difficult to prepare meals. Those who live alone and are isolated are more at risk. Some people do not have enough money to spend on food, and others have limited cooking skills.

- Digestive disorders and stomach conditions: If the body does not absorb nutrients efficiently, even a healthful diet may not prevent malnutrition. People with Crohn's disease or ulcerative colitis may need to have part of the small intestine removed to enable them to absorb nutrients.

- Celiac disease is a genetic disorder that involves a gluten intolerance. It may result in damage to the lining of the intestines and poor food absorption.

- Persistent diarrhea, vomiting, or both can lead to a loss of vital nutrients.

- Alcoholism: Addiction to alcohol can lead to gastritis or damage to the pancreas. These can make it hard to digest food, absorb certain vitamins, and produce hormones that regulate metabolism.

- Alcohol contains calories, so the person may not feel hungry. They may not eat enough proper food to supply the body with essential nutrients.

- Lack of breastfeeding: Not breastfeeding, especially in the developing world, can lead to malnutrition in infants and children.

## Risk Factors

In some parts of the world, widespread and long-term malnutrition can result from a lack of food.

In the wealthier nations, those most at risk of malnutrition are:

- Older people, especially those who are hospitalized or in long-term institutional care.

- Individuals who are socially isolated.

- People on low incomes.

- Those who have difficulty absorbing nutrients.

- People with chronic eating disorders, such as bulimia or anorexia nervosa.

- People who are recovering from a serious illness or condition.

## Diagnosis

Prompt diagnosis and treatment can prevent the development and complications of malnutrition.

There are several ways to identify adults who are malnourished or at risk of malnutrition, for example, the Malnutrition Universal Screening Tool (MUST) tool. Must have been designed to identify adults, and especially older people, with malnourishment or a high risk of malnutrition.

It is a 5-step plan that can help health care providers diagnose and treat these conditions.

Here are the steps:

- Step 1: Measure height and weight, calculate body mass index (BMI), and provide a score.

- Step 2: Note the percentage of unplanned weight loss and provide a score. For example, an unplanned loss of 5 to 10 percent of weight would give a score of 1, but a 10-percent loss would score 2.

- Step 3: Identify any mental or physical health condition and score. For example, if a person has been acutely ill and taken no food for over 5 days, the score will be 3.

- Step 4: Add scores from steps 1, 2 and 3 to obtain an overall risk score.

- Step 5: Use local guidelines to develop a care plan.

If the person is at low risk of malnutrition, their overall score will be 0. A score of 1 denotes a medium risk and 2 or more indicates a high risk.

MUST is only used to identify malnutrition or the risk of malnutrition in adults. It will not identify specific nutritional imbalances or deficiences.

## Treatment

Following the must screening, the following may happen:

- Low risk: Recommendations include ongoing screening at the hospital and at home.

- Medium risk: The person may undergo observation, their dietary intake will be documented for 3 days, and they will receive ongoing screening.

- High risk: The person will need treatment from a nutritionist and possibly other specialists, and they will undergo ongoing care.

For all risk categories, help and advice on food choices and dietary habits should be offered.

## Treatment Types

The type of treatment will depend on the severity of the malnutrition, and the presence of any underlying conditions or complications.

The healthcare provider will prepare a targeted care plan, with specific aims for treatment. There will normally be a feeding program with a specially planned diet, and possibly some additional nutritional supplements. People with severe malnourishment or absorption problems may need artificial nutritional support, either through a tube or intravenously.

The patient will be closely monitored for progress, and their treatment will be regularly reviewed to ensure their nutritional needs are being met.

## Diet

A dietician will discuss healthful food choices and dietary patterns with the patient, to encourage them to consume a healthy, nutritious diet with the right number of calories. Those who are undernourished may need additional calories to start with.

## Monitoring Progress

Regular monitoring can help ensure an appropriate intake of calories and nutrients. This may be adjusted as the patient's requirements change. Patients receiving artificial nutritional support will start eating normally as soon as they can.

## Prevention

To prevent malnutrition, people need to consume a range of nutrients from a variety of food types. There should be a balanced intake of carbohydrates, fats, protein, vitamins and minerals, as well as plenty of fluids, and especially water.

People with ulcerative colitis, Crohn's disease, celiac disease, alcoholism and other health issues will receive appropriate treatment for their condition.

# Food Processing

Food processing is the set of methods and techniques used to transform raw ingredients into food or food into other forms for consumption by humans or animals either in the home or by the food processing industry. Food processing typically takes clean, harvested crops or slaughtered and butchered animal products and uses these to produce attractive, marketable, and often long-life food products. Similar processes are used to produce animal feed. Extreme examples of food processing include the expert removal of toxic portions of the fugu fish or preparing space food for consumption under zero gravity.

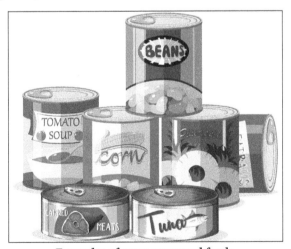
Examples of some processed foods.

The benefits of food processing include the preservation, distribution, and marketing of food, protection from pathogenic microbes and toxic substances, year-round availability of many food items, and ease of preparation by the consumer. On the other hand, food processing can lower the nutritional value of foods, and processed foods may include additives (such as colorings, flavorings, and preservatives) that may have adverse health effects.

## Food Processing Methods

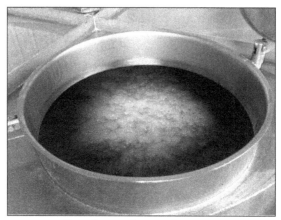

Beer fermenting at a brewery.

Common food processing techniques include:

- Removal of unwanted outer layers, such as potato peeling or the skinning of peaches.
- Chopping or slicing, such as to produce diced carrots.
- Mincing and macerating.
- Liquefaction, such as to produce fruit juice.
- Fermentation, as in beer breweries.
- Emulsification.
- Cooking, by methods such as baking, boiling, broiling, frying, steaming, or grilling.
- Mixing.
- Addition of gas such as air entrainment for bread or gasification of soft drinks.
- Proofing.
- Spray drying.
- Pasteurization.
- Packaging.

## Performance Parameters for Food Processing

When designing processes for the food industry, the following performance parameters may be taken into account:

- Hygiene, measured, for instance, by the number of microorganisms per ml of finished product.

- Energy consumption, measured, for instance, by "ton of steam per ton of sugar produced".

- Minimization of waste, measured, for instance, by the "percentage of peeling loss during the peeling of potatoes".

- Labor used, measured, for instance, by the "number of working hours per ton of finished product".

- Minimization of cleaning stops, measured, for instance, by the "number of hours between cleaning stops".

## Benefits

More and more people live in the cities far away from where food is grown and produced. In many families, the adults are work from home and therefore there is little time for the preparation of food based on fresh ingredients. The food industry offers products that fulfill many different needs: from peeled potatoes that simply need to be boiled at home to fully prepare ready meals that can be heated up in the microwave oven in a few minutes.

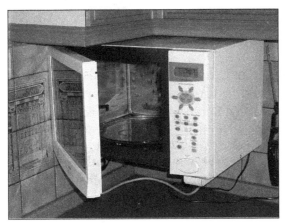
Microwave oven.

Benefits of food processing include toxin removal, preservation, easing marketing and distribution tasks and increasing food consistency. In addition, it increases seasonal availability of many foods, enables transportation of delicate perishable foods across long distances, and makes many kinds of foods safe to eat by de-activating spoilage and pathogenic micro-organisms. Modern supermarkets would not be feasible without modern food processing techniques, long voyages would not be possible, and military campaigns would be significantly more difficult and costly to execute.

Modern food processing also improves the quality of life for allergy sufferers, diabetics, and other people who cannot consume some common food elements. Food processing can also add extra nutrients such as vitamins.

Processed foods are often less susceptible to early spoilage than fresh foods, and are better suited for long distance transportation from the source to the consumer. Fresh materials, such as fresh produce and raw meats, are more likely to harbor pathogenic microorganisms (for example, Salmonella) capable of causing serious illnesses.

## Drawbacks

In general, fresh food that has not been processed other than by washing and simple kitchen preparation, may be expected to contain a higher proportion of naturally occurring vitamins, fiber and minerals than the equivalent product processed by the food industry. Vitamin C, for example, is destroyed by heat and therefore canned fruits have a lower content of vitamin C than fresh ones.

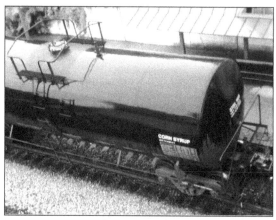
Corn syrup being moved by tank car.

Food processing can lower the nutritional value of foods. Processed foods tend to include food additives, such as flavorings and texture enhancing agents, which may have little or no nutritive value, and some may be unhealthy. Some preservatives added or created during processing, such as nitrites or sulfites, may cause adverse health effects.

Processed foods often have a higher ratio of calories to other essential nutrients than unprocessed foods, a phenomenon referred to as "empty calories." Most junk foods are processed, and fit this category.

High quality and hygiene standards must be maintained to ensure consumer safety, and failure to maintain adequate standards can have serious health consequences.

Processing food is a very costly process, thus increasing the prices of foods products.

## Trends in Modern Food Processing

## Health

- Reduction of fat content in final product, for example, by using baking instead of deep-frying in the production of potato chips.

- Maintaining the natural taste of the product, for example, by using less artificial sweetener.

## Hygiene

The rigorous application of industry and government endorsed standards to minimize possible risk and hazards. In the U.S., the standard adopted is HACCP.

## Efficiency

- Rising energy costs lead to increasing usage of energy-saving technologies, for example, frequency converters on electrical drives, heat insulation of factory buildings, and heated vessels, energy recovery systems.

- Factory automation systems (often Distributed control systems) reduce personnel costs and may lead to more stable production results.

## References

- What-food-science, foodscience: mcgill.ca, Retrieved 05 March, 2019

- Nutrition, science: britannica.com, Retrieved 23 July, 2019

- Human-nutrition, science: britannica.com, Retrieved 15 June, 2019

- Food-processing, entry: newworldencyclopedia.org, Retrieved 28 February, 2019

# 2
# Branches of Food Science

The field of food science can be branched into 4 major divisions. It includes food chemistry, food engineering, food technology and food microbiology. This chapter has been carefully written to provide an easy understanding of these branches of food science.

## Food Chemistry

Food chemistry is the study of chemical processes and interactions of the biological and nonbiological components of foods. It overlaps with biochemistry in that it deals with the components of food such as carbohydrates, lipids, proteins, water, vitamins, and dietary minerals. In addition, it involves the study and development of food additives that can be used to preserve the quality of food or to modify its color, flavor and taste. It is, thus, closely linked to food processing and preparation techniques. There is, however, an ongoing debate about the health effects of a number of food additives.

The molecular structure of sucrose, or ordinary table sugar.
This sugar is probably the most familiar carbohydrate.

### Water

A major component of food is water, which can range in content from 50 percent in meat products to 95 percent in lettuce, cabbage, and tomato products. It also provides a place for bacterial growth and food spoilage if it is not properly processed. One way of measuring this in food is by water activity, which is very important in the shelf life of many foods during processing. One of the keys to food preservation is to reduce the amount of water or alter the water's characteristics to enhance shelf-life. Such methods include dehydration, freezing, and refrigeration.

## Carbohydrates

Carbohydrates form the largest group of substances in food consumed by humans. A common carbohydrate is starch. The simplest version of a carbohydrate is a monosaccharide, made up of molecules in which carbon, hydrogen, and oxygen atoms are in the ratio 1:2:1. Thus, the general formula of a monosaccharide is $C_nH_{2n}O_n$, where n is a minimum of 3. Glucose and fructose are examples of monosaccharides. The familiar table sugar is sucrose, a disaccharide. Each molecule of sucrose is made up of a combination of one glucose and one fructose molecule.

A chain of monosaccharides forms a polysaccharide. Such polysaccharides include pectin, dextran, agar and xanthan.

Sugar content is commonly measured in degrees brix.

## Lipids

The term lipid encompasses a diverse range of molecules and to some extent is a catchall for relatively water-insoluble (nonpolar) compounds of biological origin. Examples of lipids are waxes, fatty acids, fatty-acid derived phospholipids, sphingolipids, glycolipids, and terpenoids, such as retinoids and steroids. Some lipids are linear aliphatic molecules, while others have ring structures. Some are aromatic. Some are flexible, and others are rigid.

Most lipids have some polar character, in addition to being largely nonpolar. In other words, the bulk of the structure of a lipid molecule is nonpolar or hydrophobic, meaning that it does not interact well with polar solvents like water. Another part of the molecular structure is polar or hydrophilic and will tend to associate with polar solvents like water. Thus lipid molecules are amphiphilic, having both hydrophobic and hydrophilic portions. In the case of cholesterol, the polar group is a mere -OH (hydroxyl or alcohol).

In food, lipids are present in the oils of grains such as corn and soybean, and they are also found in meat, milk, and dairy products. They act as vitamin carriers as well.

## Proteins

Proteins make up over 50 percent of the dry weight of an average living cell and are very complex macromolecules. They play a fundamental role in the structure and function of cells. Protein molecules are constructed mainly of carbon, hydrogen, oxygen, and some sulfur, they may also contain iron, copper, phosphorus, or zinc.

In food, proteins are essential for growth and survival, but the amount of protein needed by an individual varies, based on the person's age and physiology (such as during pregnancy). Proteins in food are commonly found in peanuts, meat, poultry, and seafood.

## Enzymes

Many proteins are enzymes that catalyze biochemical reactions. They reduce the amount of time and energy required to complete the reactions. Many areas of the food industry use enzyme catalysts, including baking, brewing, and dairy, to make bread, beer, and cheese.

## Vitamins

Riboflavin (Vitamin B$_2$) is a water-soluble vitamin.

Vitamins are nutrients required in small amounts for essential metabolic reactions in the body. They are subdivided as either water-soluble (such as Vitamin C) or fat-soluble (such as Vitamin E). An adequate supply of vitamins can prevent such diseases as beriberi, anemia, and scurvy, but an overdose of vitamins can produce nausea and vomiting or even death.

## Minerals

Dietary minerals in foods are large and diverse, with many required for health and survival. Some minerals, however, can be hazardous if consumed in excessive amounts. Bulk minerals with a Reference Daily Intake (RDI; formerly, Recommended Daily Allowance (RDA)) of more than 200 mg/ day include calcium, magnesium, and potassium. Important trace minerals, with RDI less than 200 mg/day, include copper, iron, and zinc. They are found in many foods but can also be taken in dietary supplements.

## Food additives

Food additives are substances added to food for such purposes as preserving its quality, adding to or enhancing its flavors, improving its taste, or modifying its appearance. Additives used today can be placed in a wide range of groups, such as food acids, anticaking agents, antioxidants, bulking agents, food coloring, flavoring agents, humectants, preservatives, stabilizers, and thickeners. They are generally listed by "E number" in the European Union or GRAS ("Generally recognized as safe") by the United States Food and Drug Administration.

## Coloring

Food coloring is added to change or enhance the color of any food, mainly to make it look more appealing. It can be used to simulate the natural color of a product as perceived by the customer, such as adding the red dye FD&C Red No.40 (Allura Red AC) to ketchup. Alternatively, unnatural colors may be added to a product like Kellogg's Fruit Loops. Caramel is a natural food dye; the industrial form, caramel coloring, is the most widely used food coloring and is found in foods ranging from soft drinks to soy sauce, bread and pickles.

## Flavors

Flavor in food is important in determining how food smells and tastes to the consumer, especially in sensory analysis. Some of these products occur naturally, such as salt and sugar, but flavor chemists (called "flavorists") develop many flavors for food products. Such artificial flavors include methyl salicylate, which produces the wintergreen odor and lactic acid, which gives milk a tart taste.

## Food Engineering

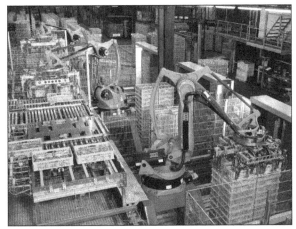

Bread factory in Germany.

Food engineering is a multidisciplinary field which combines microbiology, applied physical sciences, chemistry and engineering for food and related industries. Food engineering includes, but is not limited to, the application of agricultural engineering, mechanical engineering and chemical engineering principles to food materials. Food engineers provide the technological knowledge transfer essential to the cost-effective production and commercialization of food products and services. Physics, chemistry, and mathematics are fundamental to understanding and engineering products and operations in the food industry.

Food engineering encompasses a wide range of activities. Food engineers are employed in food processing, food machinery, packaging, ingredient manufacturing, instrumentation, and control. Firms that design and build food processing plants, consulting firms, government agencies, pharmaceutical companies, and health-care firms also employ food engineers. Specific food engineering activities include:

- Drug/food products.
- Design and installation of food/biological/pharmaceutical production processes.
- Design and operation of environmentally responsible waste treatment systems.
- Marketing and technical support for manufacturing plants.

In the development of food engineering, one of the many challenges is to employ modern tools, technology, and knowledge, such as computational materials science and nanotechnology, to develop new products and processes. Simultaneously, improving quality, safety, and security remain critical issues in food engineering study. New packaging materials and techniques are being developed to provide more protection to foods, and novel preservation technology is emerging. Additionally, process control and automation regularly appear among the top priorities identified in food engineering. Advanced monitoring and control systems are developed to facilitate automation and flexible food manufacturing. Furthermore, energy saving and minimization of environmental problems continue to be important food engineering issues, and significant progress is being made in waste management, efficient utilization of energy, and reduction of effluents and emissions in food production.

Typical topics include:

- Advances in classical unit operations in engineering applied to food manufacturing.

- Progresses in the transport and storage of liquid and solid foods.

- Developments in heating, chilling and freezing of foods.

- Advanced mass transfer in foods.

- Advances in cleaning and sanitation.

- Low moisture content foods.

- New chemical and biochemical aspects of food engineering and the use of kinetic analysis.

- Process design and development of various alternative nonthermal food preservation methods using lethal agents such as high pressure, pulsed electric field, UV, ultrasound, ozone and cold plasma.

- New techniques in dehydration, thermal processing, extrusion, liquid food concentration, membrane processes and applications of membranes in food processing.

- Shelf-life, electronic indicators in inventory management, and sustainable technologies in food processing.

- Modern packaging, cleaning, and sanitation technologies.

- Development of sensors systems for quality and safety assessment.

# Food Technology

Food technology is a branch of food science that deals with the production processes that make foods.

Early scientific research into food technology concentrated on food preservation. Nicolas Appert's development in 1810 of the canning process was a decisive event. The process wasn't called canning then and Appert did not really know the principle on which his process worked, but canning has had a major impact on food preservation techniques.

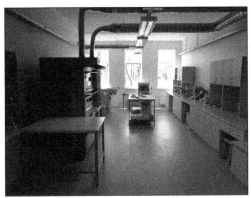 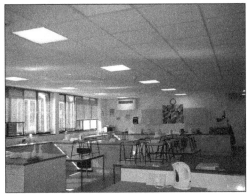

Bakery at the Faculty of Food Technology, Latvia University of Life Sciences and Technologies.

The food technology room at Marling School in Stroud, Gloucestershire.

Louis Pasteur's research on the spoilage of wine and his description of how to avoid spoilage in 1864 was an early attempt to apply scientific knowledge to food handling. Besides research into wine spoilage, Pasteur researched the production of alcohol, vinegar, wines and beer, and the souring of milk. He developed pasteurization—the process of heating milk and milk products to destroy food spoilage and disease-producing organisms. In his research into food technology, Pasteur became the pioneer into bacteriology and of modern preventive medicine.

## Developments

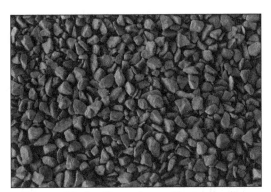

Freeze-dried coffee, a form of instant coffee.

Developments in food technology have contributed greatly to the food supply and have changed our world. Some of these developments are:

- Instantized Milk Powder: D.D. Peebles (U.S. patent 2,835,586) developed the first instant milk powder, which has become the basis for a variety of new products that are rehydratable. This process increases the surface area of the powdered product by partially rehydrating spray-dried milk powder.

- Freeze-drying: The first application of freeze drying was most likely in the pharmaceutical industry; however, a successful large-scale industrial application of the process was the development of continuous freeze drying of coffee.

- High-Temperature Short Time Processing: These processes, for the most part, are characterized by rapid heating and cooling, holding for a short time at a relatively high temperature and filling aseptically into sterile containers.

- Decaffeination of Coffee and Tea: Decaffeinated coffee and tea was first developed on a commercial basis in Europe around 1900. The process is described in U.S. patent 897,763. Green coffee beans are treated with water, heat and solvents to remove the caffeine from the beans.

- Process optimization: Food Technology now allows production of foods to be more efficient, Oil saving technologies are now available on different forms. Production methods and methodology have also become increasingly sophisticated.

## Consumer Acceptance

Historically, consumers paid little attention to food technologies. Nowadays the food production chain is long and complicated, and foods and food technologies are diverse. Consequently consumers are uncertain about the determinants of food quality and safety and find it difficult to understand them. Now, acceptance of food products very often depends on perceived benefits and risks associated with the food. Popular views of food processing technologies matter. Especially innovative food processing technologies often are perceived as risky by consumers.

Acceptance of the different food technologies varies. While pasteurization is well recognized and accepted, high pressure treatment and even microwaves often are perceived as risky. Studies by the Hightech Europe project found that traditional technologies were well accepted in contrast to innovative technologies.

Consumers form their attitude towards innovative food technologies through three main mechanisms: First, through knowledge or beliefs about risks and benefits correlated with the technology; second, through attitudes based on their own experience; and third, through application of higher order values and beliefs. A number of scholars consider the risk-benefit trade-off as one of the main determinants of consumer acceptance, although some researchers place more emphasis on the role of benefit perception (rather than risk) in consumer acceptance.

Rogers defines five major criteria that explain differences in the acceptance of new technology by consumers: complexity, compatibility, relative advantage, trialability and observability.

Acceptance of innovative technologies can be improved by providing non-emotional and concise information about these new technological processes methods. The HighTech project also suggests that written information has a higher impact on consumers than audio-visual information.

## Food Microbiology

Food microbiology is the study of the microorganisms that inhibit, create, or contaminate food, including the study of microorganisms causing food spoilage, pathogens that may cause disease especially if food is improperly cooked or stored, those used to produce fermented foods such as cheese, yogurt, bread, beer, and wine, and those with other useful roles such as producing probiotics.

## Food Safety

Food safety is a major focus of food microbiology. Numerous agents of disease, pathogens, are readily transmitted via food, including bacteria, and viruses. Microbial toxins are also possible contaminants of food. However, microorganisms and their products can also be used to combat these pathogenic microbes. Probiotic bacteria, including those that produce bacteriocins, can kill and inhibit pathogens. Alternatively, purified bacteriocins such as nisin can be added directly to food products. Finally, bacteriophages, viruses that only infect bacteria, can be used to kill bacterial pathogens. Thorough preparation of food, including proper cooking, eliminates most bacteria and viruses. However, toxins produced by contaminants may not be liable to change to non-toxic forms by heating or cooking the contaminated food due to other safety conditions.

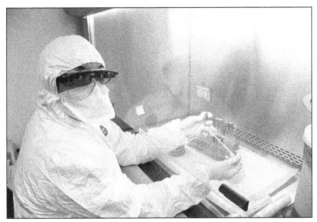

A microbiologist working in a biosafety laboratory
tests for high risk pathogens in food.

## Fermentation

Fermentation is one of the methods to preserve food and alter its quality. Yeast, especially Saccharomyces cerevisiae, is used to leaven bread, brew beer and make wine. Certain bacteria, including lactic acid bacteria, are used to make yogurt, cheese, hot sauce, pickles, fermented sausages and dishes such as kimchi. A common effect of these fermentations is that the food product is less hospitable to other microorganisms, including pathogens and spoilage-causing microorganisms, thus extending the food's shelf-life. Some cheese varieties also require molds to ripen and develop their characteristic flavors.

## Microbial Biopolymers

Several microbially produced biopolymers are used in the food industry.

- Alginate: Alginates can be used as thickening agents. commercial alginates are currently only produced by extraction from brown seaweeds such as Laminaria hyperborea or L. japonica.

- Poly-γ-glutamic acid: Poly-γ-glutamic acid (γ-PGA) produced by various strains of *Bacillus* has potential applications as a thickener in the food industry.

## Food Testing

To ensure safety of food products, microbiological tests such as testing for pathogens and spoilage organisms are required. This way the risk of contamination under normal use conditions can be examined and food poisoning outbreaks can be prevented. Testing of food products and ingredients is important along the whole supply chain as possible flaws of products can occur at every stage of production. Apart from detecting spoilage, microbiological tests can also determine germ content, identify yeasts and molds, and salmonella. For salmonella, scientists are also developing rapid and portable technologies capable of identifying unique variants of Salmonella.

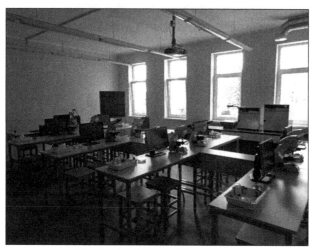

Food microbiology laboratory.

Polymerase Chain Reaction (PCR) is a quick and inexpensive method to generate numbers of copies of a DNA fragment at a specific band ("PCR (Polymerase Chain Reaction)," 2008). For that reason, scientists are using PCR to detect different kinds of viruses or bacteria, such as HIV and anthrax based on their unique DNA patterns. Various kits are commercially available to help in food pathogen nucleic acids extraction, PCR detection, and differentiation. The detection of bacterial strands in food products is very important to everyone in the world, for it helps prevent the occurrence of food borne illness. Therefore, PCR is recognized as a DNA detector in order to amplify and trace the presence of pathogenic strands in different processed food.

## References

- Food-chemistry, entry: newworldencyclopedia.org, Retrieved 25 July, 2019

- Singh, R Paul; Dennis R. Heldman (2013). Introduction to Food Engineering (5th ed.). Academic Press. p. 1. ISBN 978-0123985309

- Frewer, Lynn J.; van der Lans, Ivo A.; Fischer, Arnout R.H.; Reinders, Machiel J.; Menozzi, Davide; Zhang, Xiaoyong; van den Berg, Isabelle; Zimmermann, Karin L. (April 2013). "Public perceptions of agri-food applications of genetic modification – A systematic review and meta-analysis". Trends in Food Science & Technology. 30 (2): 142–152. doi:10.1016/j.tifs.2013.01.003

- Fratamico PM (2005). Bayles DO (ed.). Foodborne Pathogens: Microbiology and Molecular Biology. Caister Academic Press. ISBN 978-1-904455-00-4

# 3

# Nutrients

The nutrients can be broadly classified into two categories, namely, micronutrients and macronutrients. Some of the micronutrients are vitamins and minerals while carbohydrates, proteins and fats fall under macronutrients. This chapter discusses about these different types of essential nutrients in detail.

## Carbohydrates

Carbohydrates are the sugars, starches and fibers found in fruits, grains, vegetables and milk products. Though often maligned in trendy diets, carbohydrates — one of the basic food groups are important to a healthy diet.

"Carbohydrates are macronutrients, meaning they are one of the three main ways the body obtains energy or calories". The American Diabetes Association notes that carbohydrates are the body's main source of energy. They are called carbohydrates because, at the chemical level, they contain carbon, hydrogen and oxygen.

There are three macronutrients: carbohydrates, protein and fats. Macronutrients are essential for proper body functioning, and the body requires large amounts of them. All macronutrients must be obtained through diet; the body cannot produce macronutrients on its own.

The recommended daily amount (RDA) of carbs for adults is 135 grams Carb intake for most people should be between 45% and 65% of total calories. One gram of carbohydrates equals about 4 calories, so a diet of 1,800 calories per day would equal about 202 grams on the low end and 292 gram of carbs on the high end. However, people with diabetes should not eat more than 200 grams of carbs per day, while pregnant women need at least 175 grams.

### Function of Carbohydrates

Carbohydrates provide fuel for the central nervous system and energy for working muscles. They also prevent protein from being used as an energy source and enable fat metabolism.

Also, "carbohydrates are important for brain function". They are an influence on "mood, memory, etc., as well as a quick energy source." In fact, the RDA of carbohydrates is based on the amount of carbs the brain needs to function.

Two recent studies have also linked carbs to decision-making. In the studies, people who ate a high-carbohydrate breakfast were less willing to share when playing the "ultimatum game" than those who ate high-protein breakfasts. Scientists speculate this may be caused by baseline dopamine levels, which are higher after eating carbohydrates. This doesn't mean carbs make you mean, but underscores how different types of food intake can affect cognition and behavior.

## Simple versus Complex Carbohydrates

Carbohydrates are classified as simple or complex. The difference between the two forms is the chemical structure and how quickly the sugar is absorbed and digested. Generally speaking, simple carbs are digested and absorbed more quickly and easily than complex carbs.

Simple carbohydrates contain just one or two sugars, such as fructose (found in fruits) and galactose (found in milk products). These single sugars are called monosaccharides. Carbs with two sugars such as sucrose (table sugar), lactose (from dairy) and maltose (found in beer and some vegetables) are called disaccharides.

Simple carbs are also in candy, soda and syrups. However, these foods are made with processed and refined sugars and do not have vitamins, minerals or fiber. They are called "empty calories" and can lead to weight gain.

Complex carbohydrates (polysaccharides) have three or more sugars. They are often referred to as starchy foods and include beans, peas, lentils, peanuts, potatoes, corn, parsnips, whole-grain breads and cereals.

Smathers pointed out that, while all carbohydrates function as relatively quick energy sources, simple carbs cause bursts of energy much more quickly than complex carbs because of the quicker rate at which they are digested and absorbed. Simple carbs can lead to spikes in blood sugar levels and sugar highs, while complex carbs provide more sustained energy.

Studies have shown that replacing saturated fats with simple carbs, such as those in many processed foods, is associated with an increased risk of heart disease and type 2 diabetes.

## Sugars, Starches and Fibers

In the body, carbs break down into smaller units of sugar, such as glucose and fructose. The small intestine absorbs these smaller units, which then enter the bloodstream and travel to the liver. The liver converts all of these sugars into glucose, which is carried through the bloodstream — accompanied by insulin — and converted into energy for basic body functioning and physical activity.

If the glucose is not immediately needed for energy, the body can store up to 2,000 calories of it in the liver and skeletal muscles in the form of glycogen. Once glycogen stores are full, carbs are stored as fat. If you have insufficient carbohydrate intake or stores, the body will consume protein for fuel. This is problematic because the body needs protein to make muscles. Using protein instead of carbohydrates for fuel also puts stress on the kidneys, leading to the passage of painful byproducts in the urine.

Fiber is essential to digestion. Fibers promote healthy bowel movements and decrease the risk of chronic diseases such as coronary heart disease and diabetes. However, unlike sugars and starches, fibers are not absorbed in the small intestine and are not converted to glucose. Instead, they pass into the large intestine relatively intact, where they are converted to hydrogen and carbon dioxide and fatty acids. The Institute of Medicine recommends that people consume 14 grams of fiber for every 1,000 calories. Sources of fiber include fruits, grains and vegetables, especially legumes.

Smathers pointed out that carbs are also found naturally in some forms of dairy and both starchy and nonstarchy vegetables. For example, nonstarchy vegetables like lettuces, kale, green beans, celery, carrots and broccoli all contain carbs. Starchy vegetables like potatoes and corn also contain carbohydrates, but in larger amounts. Nonstarchy vegetables generally contain only about 5 grams of carbohydrates per cup of raw vegetables, and most of those carbs come from fiber.

## Good Carbs versus Bad Carbs

Carbohydrates are found in foods you know are good for you (vegetables) and ones you know are not (doughnuts). This has led to the idea that some carbs are "good" and some are "bad." Carbs commonly considered bad include pastries, sodas, highly processed foods, white rice, white bread and other white-flour foods. These are foods with simple carbs. Bad carbs rarely have any nutritional value.

Carbs usually considered good are complex carbs, such as whole grains, fruits, vegetables, beans and legumes. These are not only processed more slowly, but they also contain a bounty of other nutrients.

Good carbs are:

- Low or moderate in calories.

- High in nutrients.

- Devoid of refined sugars and refined grains.

- High in naturally occurring fiber.

- Low in sodium.

- Low in saturated fat.

- Very low in, or devoid of, cholesterol and trans fats.

Bad carbs are:

- High in calories.

- Full of refined sugars, like corn syrup, white sugar, honey and fruit juices.

- High in refined grains like white flour.

- Low in many nutrients.

- Low in fiber.

- High in sodium.

- Sometimes high in saturated fat.

- Sometimes high in cholesterol and trans fats.

## Glycemic Index

Recently, nutritionists have said that it's not the type of carbohydrate, but rather the carb's glycemic index, that's important. The glycemic index measures how quickly and how much a carbohydrate raises blood sugar.

High-glycemic foods like pastries raise blood sugar highly and rapidly; low-glycemic foods raise it gently and to a lesser degree. Some research has linked high-glycemic foods with diabetes, obesity, heart disease and certain cancers.

On the other hand, recent research suggests that following a low-glycemic diet may not actually be helpful. A 2014 study found that overweight adults eating a balanced diet did not see much additional improvement on a low-calorie, low-glycemic index diet. Scientists measured insulin sensitivity, systolic blood pressure, LDL cholesterol and HDL cholesterol and saw that the low-glycemic diet did not improve them. It did lower triglycerides.

## Carbohydrate Benefits

The right kind of carbs can be incredibly good for you. Not only are they necessary for your health, but they carry a variety of added benefits.

## Mental Health

Carbohydrates may be important to mental health. A study found that people on a high-fat, low-carb diet for a year had more anxiety, depression and anger than people on a low-fat, high-carb diet. Scientists suspect that carbohydrates help with the production of serotonin in the brain.

Carbs may help memory, too. A 2008 study had overweight women cut carbs entirely from their diets for one week. Then, they tested the women's cognitive skills, visual attention and spatial memory. The women on no-carb diets did worse than overweight women on low-calorie diets that contained a healthy amount of carbohydrates.

## Weight Loss

Though carbs are often blamed for weight gain, the right kind of carbs can actually help you lose and maintain a healthy weight. This happens because many good carbohydrates, especially whole grains and vegetables with skin, contain fiber. It is difficult to get sufficient fiber on a low-carb diet. Dietary fiber helps you to feel full, and generally comes in relatively low-calorie foods.

A study followed middle-age women for 20 months and found that participants who ate more fiber lost weight, while those who decreased their fiber intake gained weight. Another recent study linked fat loss with low-fat diets, not low-carb ones.

While some studies have found that low-carb diets do help people lose weight, a meta-analysis found that when viewed long term, low-fat and low-carb diets had similar success rates. People lost more weight early on while on low-carb diets but after a year they were all in similar places.

## Good Source of Nutrients

Whole, unprocessed fruits and vegetables are well known for their nutrient content. Some are even considered superfoods because of it — and all of these leafy greens, bright sweet potatoes, juicy berries, tangy citruses and crunchy apples contain carbs.

One important, plentiful source of good carbs is whole grains. A large study found that those eating the most whole grains had significantly higher amounts of fiber, energy and polyunsaturated fats, as well as all micronutrients (except vitamin B12 and sodium). An additional study, found that whole grains contain antioxidants, which were previously thought to exist almost exclusively in fruits and vegetables.

## Heart Health

Fiber also helps to lower cholesterol. The digestive process requires bile acids, which are made partly with cholesterol. As your digestion improves, the liver pulls cholesterol from the blood to create more bile acid, thereby reducing the amount of LDL, the "bad" cholesterol.

Toups referenced a study looked at the effect of whole grains on patients taking cholesterol-lowering medications called statins. Those who ate more than 16 grams of whole grains daily had lower bad-cholesterol levels than those who took the statins without eating the whole grains.

## Carbohydrate Deficiency

Not getting enough carbs can cause problems. Without sufficient fuel, the body gets no energy. Additionally, without sufficient glucose, the central nervous system suffers, which may cause dizziness or mental and physical weakness. A deficiency of glucose, or low blood sugar, is called hypoglycemia.

If the body has insufficient carbohydrate intake or stores, it will consume protein for fuel. This is problematic because the body needs protein to make muscles. Using protein for fuel instead of carbohydrates also puts stress on the kidneys, leading to the passage of painful byproducts in the urine.

People who don't consume enough carbohydrates may also suffer from insufficient fiber, which can cause digestive problems and constipation.

# Proteins

Proteins are essential nutrients for the human body. They are one of the building blocks of body tissue and can also serve as a fuel source. As a fuel, proteins provide as much energy density as carbohydrates: 4 kcal (17 kJ) per gram; in contrast, lipids provide 9 kcal (37 kJ) per gram. The most important aspect and defining characteristic of protein from a nutritional standpoint is its amino acid composition.

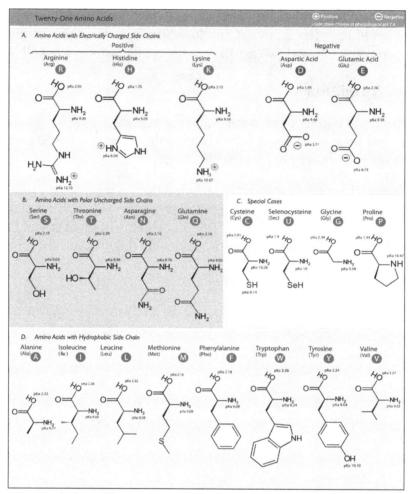

Amino acids are necessary nutrients. Present in every cell,
they are also precursors to nucleic acids, co-enzymes, hormones,
immune response, repair and other molecules essential for life.

Proteins are polymer chains made of amino acids linked together by peptide bonds. During human digestion, proteins are broken down in the stomach to smaller polypeptide chains via hydrochloric acid and protease actions. This is crucial for the absorption of the essential amino acids that cannot be biosynthesized by the body.

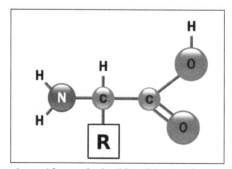

Amino acids are the building blocks of protein.

There are nine essential amino acids which humans must obtain from their diet in order to prevent protein-energy malnutrition and resulting death. They are phenylalanine, valine, threonine, tryptophan, methionine, leucine, isoleucine, lysine, and histidine. There has been debate as to whether there are 8 or 9 essential amino acids. The consensus seems to lean towards 9 since histidine is not synthesized in adults. There are five amino acids which humans are able to synthesize in the body. These five are alanine, aspartic acid, asparagine, glutamic acid and serine. There are six conditionally essential amino acids whose synthesis can be limited under special pathophysiological conditions, such as prematurity in the infant or individuals in severe catabolic distress. These six are arginine, cysteine, glycine, glutamine, proline and tyrosine.

Dietary sources of protein include both animals and plants: meats, dairy products, fish and eggs, as well as grains, legumes and nuts. Vegans can get enough essential amino acids by eating plant proteins.

## Protein Functions in the Human Body

Protein is a nutrient needed by the human body for growth and maintenance. Aside from water, proteins are the most abundant kind of molecules in the body. Protein can be found in all cells of the body and is the major structural component of all cells in the body, especially muscle. This also includes body organs, hair and skin. Proteins are also used in membranes, such as glycoproteins. When broken down into amino acids, they are used as precursors to nucleic acid, co-enzymes, hormones, immune response, cellular repair, and other molecules essential for life. Additionally, protein is needed to form blood cells.

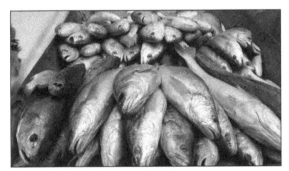
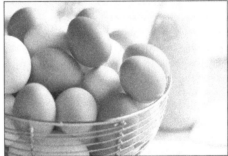
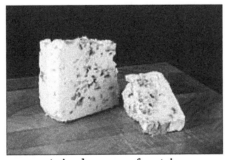

Animal sources of protein.

Protein can be found in a wide range of food. The best combination of protein sources depends on the region of the world, access, cost, amino acid types and nutrition balance, as well as acquired tastes. Some foods are high in certain amino acids, but their digestibility and the anti-nutritional factors present in these foods make them of limited value in human nutrition. Therefore, one must consider digestibility and secondary nutrition profile such as calories, cholesterol, vitamins and essential mineral density of the protein source. On a worldwide basis, plant protein foods contribute over 60 percent of the per capita supply of protein, on average. In North America, animal-derived foods contribute about 70 percent of protein sources.

Meat, products from milk, eggs, soy, and fish are sources of complete protein.

Table: Nutritional value and environmental impact of animal products, compared to agriculture overall.

| Categories | Contribution of farmed animal product [%] |
|---|---|
| Calories | 18 |
| Proteins | 37 |
| Land use | 83 |
| Greenhouse gases | 58 |
| Water pollution | 57 |
| Air pollution | 56 |
| Freshwater withdrawals | 33 |

Whole grains and cereals are another source of proteins. However, these tend to be limiting in the amino acid lysine or threonine, which are available in other vegetarian sources and meats. Examples of food staples and cereal sources of protein, each with a concentration greater than 7.0%, are (in no particular order) buckwheat, oats, rye, millet, maize (corn), rice, wheat, sorghum, amaranth, and quinoa.

Vegetarian sources of proteins include legumes, nuts, seeds and fruits. Legumes, some of which are called pulses in certain parts of the world, have higher concentrations of amino acids and are more complete sources of protein than whole grains and cereals. Examples of vegetarian foods with protein concentrations greater than 7 percent include soybeans, lentils, kidney beans, white beans, mung beans, chickpeas, cowpeas, lima beans, pigeon peas, lupines, wing beans, almonds, Brazil nuts, cashews, pecans, walnuts, cotton seeds, pumpkin seeds, hemp seeds, sesame seeds, and sunflower seeds.

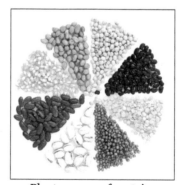

Plant sources of protein.

Food staples that are poor sources of protein include roots and tubers such as yams, cassava and sweet potato. Plantains, another major staple, are also a poor source of essential amino acids. Fruits, while rich in other essential nutrients, are another poor source of amino acids. The protein content in roots, tubers and fruits is between 0 and 2 percent. Food staples with low protein content must be complemented with foods with complete, quality protein content for a healthy life, particularly in children for proper development.

A good source of protein is often a combination of various foods, because different foods are rich in different amino acids. A good source of dietary protein meets two requirements:

- The requirement for the nutritionally indispensable amino acids (histidine, isoleucine, leucine, lysine, methionine, phenylalanine, threonine, tryptophan, and valine) under all conditions and for conditionally indispensable amino acids (cystine, tyrosine, taurine, glycine, arginine, glutamine, proline) under specific physiological and pathological conditions.

- The requirement for nonspecific nitrogen for the synthesis of the nutritionally dispensable amino acids (aspartic acid, asparagine, glutamic acid, alanine, serine) and other physiologically important nitrogen-containing compounds such as nucleic acids, creatine, and porphyrins.

Healthy people eating a balanced diet rarely need protein supplements.

The table below presents the most important food groups as protein sources, from a worldwide perspective. It also lists their respective performance as source of the commonly limiting amino acids, in milligrams of limiting amino acid per gram of total protein in the food source. The table reiterates the need for a balanced mix of foods to ensure adequate amino acid source.

| Food source | Lysine | Threonine | Tryptophan | Sulfur-containing amino acids |
|---|---|---|---|---|
| Legumes | 64 | 38 | 12 | 25 |
| Cereals and whole grains | 31 | 32 | 12 | 37 |
| Nuts and seeds | 45 | 36 | 17 | 46 |
| Fruits | 45 | 29 | 11 | 27 |
| Animal | 85 | 44 | 12 | 38 |

Protein powders – such as casein, whey, egg, rice and soy – are processed and manufactured sources of protein. These protein powders may provide an additional source of protein for bodybuilders. The type of protein is important in terms of its influence on protein metabolic response and possibly on the muscle's exercise performance. The different physical and/or chemical properties within the various types of protein may affect the rate of protein digestion. As a result, the amino acid availability and the accumulation of tissue protein is altered because of the various protein metabolic responses.

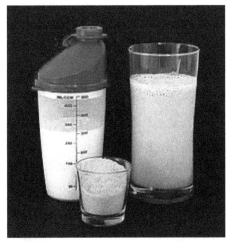

Protein milkshakes, made from protein powder (center)
and milk (left), are a common bodybuilding supplement.

## Testing in Foods

The classic assays for protein concentration in food are the Kjeldahl method and the Dumas method. These tests determine the total nitrogen in a sample. The only major component of most food which contains nitrogen is protein (fat, carbohydrate and dietary fiber do not contain nitrogen). If the amount of nitrogen is multiplied by a factor depending on the kinds of protein expected in the food the total protein can be determined. This value is known as the "*crude protein*" content. On food labels the protein is given by the nitrogen multiplied by 6.25, because the average nitrogen content of proteins is about 16%. The Kjeldahl test is typically used because it is the method the AOAC International has adopted and is therefore used by many food standards agencies around the world, though the Dumas method is also approved by some standards organizations.

Accidental contamination and intentional adulteration of protein meals with non-protein nitrogen sources that inflate crude protein content measurements have been known to occur in the food industry for decades. To ensure food quality, purchasers of protein meals routinely conduct quality control tests designed to detect the most common non-protein nitrogen contaminants, such as urea and ammonium nitrate.

In at least one segment of the food industry, the dairy industry, some countries (at least the U.S., Australia, France and Hungary) have adopted "*true protein*" measurement, as opposed to crude protein measurement, as the standard for payment and testing: "True protein is a measure of only the proteins in milk, whereas crude protein is a measure of all sources of nitrogen and includes nonprotein nitrogen, such as urea, which has no food value to humans. Current milk-testing equipment measures peptide bonds, a direct measure of true protein." Measuring peptide bonds in grains has also been put into practice in several countries including Canada, the UK, Australia, Russia and Argentina where near-infrared reflectance (NIR) technology, a type of infrared spectroscopy is used. The Food and Agriculture Organization of the United Nations (FAO) recommends that only amino acid analysis be used to determine protein in, *inter alia*, foods used as the sole source of nourishment, such as infant formula, but also provides: "When data on amino acids analyses are not available, determination of protein based on total N content by Kjeldahl (AOAC, 2000) or similar method is considered acceptable."

The testing method for protein in beef cattle feed has grown into a science over the post-war years. The standard text in the United States, Nutrient Requirements of Beef Cattle, has been through eight editions over at least seventy years. The 1996 sixth edition substituted for the fifth edition's crude protein the concept of "metabolizeable protein", which was defined around the year 2000 as "the true protein absorbed by the intestine, supplied by microbial protein and undegraded intake protein".

The limitations of the Kjeldahl method were at the heart of the Chinese protein export contamination in 2007 and the 2008 China milk scandal in which the industrial chemical melamine was added to the milk or glutens to increase the measured "protein".

## Protein Quality

The most important aspect and defining characteristic of protein from a nutritional standpoint is its amino acid composition. There are multiple systems which rate proteins by their usefulness to an organism based on their relative percentage of amino acids and, in some systems, the digestibility of the protein source. They include biological value, net protein utilization, and PDCAAS (Protein Digestibility Corrected Amino Acids Score) which was developed by the FDA as a modification of the Protein efficiency ratio (PER) method. The PDCAAS rating was adopted by the US Food and Drug Administration (FDA) and the Food and Agricultural Organization of the United Nations/World Health Organization (FAO/WHO) in 1993 as "the preferred 'best'" method to determine protein quality. These organizations have suggested that other methods for evaluating the quality of protein are inferior. In 2013 FAO proposed changing to Digestible Indispensable Amino Acid Score.

## Digestion

Most proteins are decomposed to single amino acids by digestion in the gastro-intestinal tract.

Digestion typically begins in the stomach when pepsinogen is converted to pepsin by the action of hydrochloric acid, and continued by trypsin and chymotrypsin in the small intestine. Before the absorption in the small intestine, most proteins are already reduced to single amino acid or peptides of several amino acids. Most peptides longer than four amino acids are not absorbed. Absorption into the intestinal absorptive cells is not the end. There, most of the peptides are broken into single amino acids.

Absorption of the amino acids and their derivatives into which dietary protein is degraded is done by the gastrointestinal tract. The absorption rates of individual amino acids are highly dependent on the protein source; for example, the digestibilities of many amino acids in humans, the difference between soy and milk proteins and between individual milk proteins, beta-lactoglobulin and casein. For milk proteins, about 50% of the ingested protein is absorbed between the stomach and the jejunum and 90% is absorbed by the time the digested food reaches the ileum. Biological value (BV) is a measure of the proportion of absorbed protein from a food which becomes incorporated into the proteins of the organism's body.

## Newborn

Newborns of mammals are exceptional in protein digestion and assimilation in that they can absorb intact proteins at the small intestine. This enables passive immunity, i.e., transfer of immunoglobulins from the mother to the newborn, via milk.

Dietary requirements: Considerable debate has taken place regarding issues surrounding protein intake requirements. The amount of protein required in a person's diet is determined in large part by overall energy intake, the body's need for nitrogen and essential amino acids, body weight and composition, rate of growth in the individual, physical activity level, the individual's energy and carbohydrate intake, and the presence of illness or injury. Physical activity and exertion as well as enhanced muscular mass increase the need for protein. Requirements are also greater during childhood for growth and development, during pregnancy, or when breastfeeding in order to nourish a baby or when the body needs to recover from malnutrition or trauma or after an operation.

If not enough energy is taken in through diet, as in the process of starvation, the body will use protein from the muscle mass to meet its energy needs, leading to muscle wasting over time. If the individual does not consume adequate protein in nutrition, then muscle will also waste as more vital cellular processes (e.g., respiration enzymes, blood cells) recycle muscle protein for their own requirements.

## Dietary Recommendations

According to US & Canadian Dietary Reference Intake guidelines, women aged 19–70 need to consume 46 grams of protein per day while men aged 19–70 need to consume 56 grams of protein per day to minimize risk of deficiency. These Recommended Dietary Allowances (RDAs) were calculated based on 0.8 grams protein per kilogram body weight and average body weights of 57 kg (126 pounds) and 70 kg (154 pounds), respectively. However, this recommendation is based on structural requirements but disregards use of protein for energy metabolism. This requirement is for a normal sedentary person. In the United States, average protein consumption is higher than the RDA. According to results of the National Health and Nutrition Examination Survey (NHANES 2013-2014), average protein consumption for women ages 20 and older was 69.8 grams and for men 98.3 grams/day.

## Active People

Several studies have concluded that active people and athletes may require elevated protein intake (compared to 0.8 g/kg) due to increase in muscle mass and sweat losses, as well as need for body repair and energy source. Suggested amounts vary from 1.2-1.4 g/kg for those doing endurance exercise to as much as 1.6-1.8 g/kg for strength exercise, while a proposed *maximum* daily protein intake would be approximately 25% of energy requirements i.e. approximately 2 to 2.5 g/kg. However, many questions still remain to be resolved.

In addition, some have suggested that athletes using restricted-calorie diets for weight loss should further increase their protein consumption, possibly to 1.8–2.0 g/kg, in order to avoid loss of lean muscle mass.

## Aerobic Exercise Protein Needs

Endurance athletes differ from strength-building athletes in that endurance athletes do not build as much muscle mass from training as strength-building athletes do. Research suggests that individuals performing endurance activity require more protein intake than sedentary individuals so that muscles broken down during endurance workouts can be repaired. Although the protein requirement for athletes still remains controversial, research does show that endurance athletes can benefit from increasing protein intake because the type of exercise endurance athletes participate in still alters the protein metabolism pathway. The overall protein requirement increases because of amino acid oxidation in endurance-trained athletes. Endurance athletes who exercise over a long period (2–5 hours per training session) use protein as a source of 5–10% of their total energy expended. Therefore, a slight increase in protein intake may be beneficial to endurance athletes by replacing the protein lost in energy expenditure and protein lost in repairing muscles. One review concluded that endurance athletes may increase daily protein intake to a maximum of 1.2–1.4 g per kg body weight.

## Anaerobic Exercise Protein Needs

Research also indicates that individuals performing strength-training activity require more protein than sedentary individuals. Strength-training athletes may increase their daily protein intake to a maximum of 1.4–1.8 g per kg body weight to enhance muscle protein synthesis, or to make up for the loss of amino acid oxidation during exercise. Many athletes maintain a high-protein diet as part of their training. In fact, some athletes who specialize in anaerobic sports (e.g., weightlifting) believe a very high level of protein intake is necessary, and so consume high protein meals and also protein supplements.

## Special Populations

### Protein Allergies

A food allergy is an abnormal immune response to proteins in food. The signs and symptoms may range from mild to severe. They may include itchiness, swelling of the tongue, vomiting, diarrhea, hives, trouble breathing, or low blood pressure. These symptoms typically occurs within minutes to one hour after exposure. When the symptoms are severe, it is known as anaphylaxis. The following eight foods are responsible for about 90% of allergic reactions: cow's milk, eggs, wheat, shellfish, fish, peanuts, tree nuts and soy.

### Chronic Kidney Disease

While there is no conclusive evidence that a high protein diet can cause chronic kidney disease, there is a consensus that people with this disease should decrease consumption of protein. According to one 2009 review, people with chronic kidney disease who reduce protein consumption have a 32% lower risk of death in comparison to affected people who do not make these dietary changes. Moreover, people with this disease while using a low protein diet (0.6 g/kg/d - 0.8 g/kg/d) may develop metabolic compensations that preserve kidney function, although in some people, malnutrition may occur.

### Phenylketonuria

Individuals with phenylketonuria (PKU) must keep their intake of phenylalanine - an essential amino acid - extremely low to prevent a mental disability and other metabolic complications. Phenylalanine is a component of the artificial sweetener aspartame, so people with PKU need to avoid low calorie beverages and foods with this ingredient.

### Maple Syrup Urine Disease

Maple syrup urine disease is associated with genetic anomalies in the metabolism of branched-chain amino acids (BCAAs). They have high blood levels of BCAAs and must severely restrict their intake of BCAAs in order to prevent mental retardation and death. The amino acids in question are leucine, isoleucine and valine. The condition gets its name from the distinctive sweet odor of affected infants' urine. Children of Amish, Mennonite, and Ashkenazi Jewish descent have a high prevalence of this disease compared to other populations.

### Excess Consumption

The U.S. and Canadian Dietary Reference Intake review for protein concluded that there was not sufficient evidence to establish a Tolerable upper intake level, i.e., an upper limit for how much protein can be safely consumed.

When amino acids are in excess of needs, the liver takes up the amino acids and deaminates them, a process converting the nitrogen from the amino acids into ammonia, further processed in the liver into urea via the urea cycle. Excretion of urea occurs via the kidneys. Other parts of the amino acid molecules can be converted into glucose and used for fuel. When food protein intake is periodically high or low, the body tries to keep protein levels at an equilibrium by using the "labile protein reserve" to compensate for daily variations in protein intake. However, unlike body fat as a reserve for future caloric needs, there is no protein storage for future needs.

Excessive protein intake may increase calcium excretion in urine, occurring to compensate for the pH imbalance from oxidation of sulfur amino acids. This may lead to a higher risk of kidney stone formation from calcium in the renal circulatory system. One meta-analysis reported no adverse effects of higher protein intakes on bone density. Another meta-analysis reported a small decrease in systolic and diastolic blood pressure with diets higher in protein, with no differences between animal and plant protein.

High protein diets have been shown to lead to an additional 1.21 kg of weight loss over a period of 3 months versus a baseline protein diet in a meta-analysis. Benefits of decreased body mass index as well as HDL cholesterol were more strongly observed in studies with only a slight increase in protein intake rather where high protein intake was classified as 45% of total energy intake. Detrimental effects to cardiovascular activity were not observed in short-term diets of 6 months or less. There is little consensus on the potentially detrimental effects to healthy individuals of a long-term high protein diet, leading to caution advisories about using high protein intake as a form of weight loss.

The 2015–2020 Dietary Guidelines for Americans (DGA) recommends that men and teenage boys increase their consumption of fruits, vegetables and other under-consumed foods, and that a means of accomplishing this would be to reduce overall intake of protein foods. The 2015 - 2020 DGA report does not set a recommended limit for the intake of red and processed meat. While the report acknowledges research showing that lower intake of red and processed meat is correlated with reduced risk of cardiovascular diseases in adults, it also notes the value of nutrients provided from these meats. The recommendation is not to limit intake of meats or protein, but rather to monitor and keep within daily limits the sodium (< 2300 mg), saturated fats (less than 10% of total calories per day), and added sugars (less than 10% of total calories per day) that may be increased as a result of consumption of certain meats and proteins. While the 2015 DGA report does advise for a reduced level of consumption of red and processed meats, the 2015-2020 DGA key recommendations recommend that a variety of protein foods be consumed, including both vegetarian and non-vegetarian sources of protein.

## Protein Deficiency

Protein deficiency and malnutrition (PEM) can lead to variety of ailments including mental retardation and kwashiorkor. Symptoms of kwashiorkor include apathy, diarrhea, inactivity, failure to grow, flaky skin, fatty liver, and edema of the belly and legs. This edema is explained by the action of lipoxygenase on arachidonic acid to form leukotrienes and the normal functioning of proteins in fluid balance and lipoprotein transport.

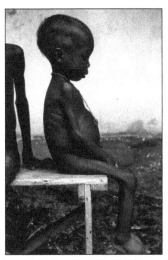

A child in Nigeria during the Biafra War suffering from
kwashiorkor – one of the three protein energy malnutrition
ailments afflicting over 10 million children in developing countries.

PEM is fairly common worldwide in both children and adults and accounts for 6 million deaths annually. In the industrialized world, PEM is predominantly seen in hospitals, is associated with disease, or is often found in the elderly.

## Fats

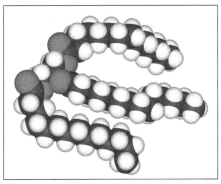

A fat, or triglyceride, molecule. Note the three fatty acid chains
attached to the central glycerol portion of the molecule.

Fats are one of the three main macronutrients, along with carbohydrates and proteins. Fat molecules consist of primarily carbon and hydrogen atoms and are therefore hydrophobic and are soluble in organic solvents and insoluble in water. Examples include cholesterol, phospholipids, and triglycerides.

The terms lipid, oil, and fat are often confused. Lipid is the general term, though a lipid is not necessarily a triglyceride. Oil normally refers to a lipid with short or unsaturated fatty acid chains that is liquid at room temperature, while fat (in the strict sense) specifically refers to lipids that are solids at room temperature – however, fat (in the broad sense) may be used in food science as a synonym for lipid.

Fat is an important foodstuff for many forms of life, and fats serve both structural and metabolic functions. They are a necessary part of the diet of most heterotrophs (including humans) and are the most energy dense, thus the most efficient form of energy storage.

Some fatty acids that are set free by the digestion of fats are called essential because they cannot be synthesized in the body from simpler constituents. There are two essential fatty acids (EFAs) in human nutrition: alpha-linolenic acid (an omega-3 fatty acid) and linoleic acid (an omega-6 fatty acid). Other lipids needed by the body can be synthesized from these and other fats. Fats and other lipids are broken down in the body by enzymes called lipases produced in the pancreas.

Fats and oils are categorized according to the number and bonding of the carbon atoms in the aliphatic chain. Fats that are saturated fats have no double bonds between the carbons in the chain. Unsaturated fats have one or more double bonded carbons in the chain. The nomenclature is based on the non-acid (non-carbonyl) end of the chain. This end is called the omega end or the n-end. Thus alpha-linolenic acid is called an omega-3 fatty acid because the 3rd carbon from that end is the first double bonded carbon in the chain counting from that end. Some oils and fats have multiple double bonds and are therefore called polyunsaturated fats. Unsaturated fats can be further divided into cis fats, which are the most common in nature, and trans fats, which are rare in nature. Unsaturated fats can be altered by reaction with hydrogen effected by a catalyst. This action, called hydrogenation, tends to break all the double bonds and makes a fully saturated fat. To make vegetable shortening, then, liquid *cis*-unsaturated fats such as vegetable oils are hydrogenated to produce saturated fats, which have more desirable physical properties e.g., they melt at a desirable temperature (30–40 °C), and store well, whereas polyunsaturated oils go rancid when they react with oxygen in the air. However, trans fats are generated during hydrogenation as contaminants created by an unwanted side reaction on the catalyst during partial hydrogenation.

Saturated fats can stack themselves in a closely packed arrangement, so they can solidify easily and are typically solid at room temperature. For example, animal fats tallow and lard are high in saturated fatty acid content and are solids. Olive and linseed oils on the other hand are unsaturated and liquid. Fats serve both as energy sources for the body, and as stores for energy in excess of what the body needs immediately. Each gram of fat when burned or metabolized releases about 9 food calories (37 kJ = 8.8 kcal). Fats are broken down in the healthy body to release their constituents, glycerol and fatty acids. Glycerol itself can be converted to glucose by the liver and so become a source of energy.

## Chemical Structure

The above figure shows the example of a natural triglyceride with three different fatty acids. One fatty acid is saturated (blue highlighted), another contains one double bond within the carbon chain (green highlighted). The third fatty acid (a polyunsaturated fatty acid, highlighted in red) contains three double bonds within the carbon chain. All carbon-carbon double bonds shown are *cis* isomers.

There are many different kinds of fats, but each is a variation on the same chemical structure. All fats are derivatives of fatty acids and glycerol. Most fats are glycerides, particularly triglycerides (triesters of glycerol). One chain of fatty acid is bonded to each of the three -OH groups of the glycerol by the reaction of the carboxyl end of the fatty acid (-COOH) with the alcohol; I.e. three chains per molecule. Water is eliminated and the carbons are linked by an -O- bond through dehydration synthesis. This process is called esterification and fats are therefore esters. As a simple visual illustration, if the kinks and angles of these chains were straightened out, the molecule would have the shape of a capital letter E. The fatty acids would each be a horizontal line; the glycerol "backbone" would be the vertical line that joins the horizontal lines. Fats therefore have "ester" bonds.

The properties of any specific fat molecule depend on the particular fatty acids that constitute it. Fatty acids form a family of compounds that are composed of increasing numbers of carbon atoms linked into a zig-zag chain (hydrogen atoms to the side). The more carbon atoms there are in any fatty acid, the longer its chain will be. Long chains are more susceptible to intermolecular forces of attraction (in this case, van der Waals forces), and so the longer ones melt at a higher temperature (melting point).

Table: Examples of fatty acids.

| Trans Unsaturated (Example shown: Elaidic acid) | Cis Unsaturated (Example shown: Oleic acid) | Saturated (Example shown: Stearic acid) |
|---|---|---|
| | | |
| Elaidic acid is the principal trans unsaturated fatty acid often found in partially hydrogenated vegetable oils. | Oleic acid is a cis unsaturated fatty acid making up 55–80% of olive oil. | Stearic acid is a saturated fatty acid found in animal fats and is the intended product in full hydrogenation. Stearic acid is neither cis nor trans because it has no carbon-carbon double bonds. |

Fatty acid chains may also differ by length, often categorized as short to very long.

- Short-chain fatty acids (SCFA) are fatty acids with aliphatic tails of fewer than six carbons (i.e. butyric acid).

- Medium-chain fatty acids (MCFA) are fatty acids with aliphatic tails of 6–12 carbons, which can form medium-chain triglycerides.

- Long-chain fatty acids (LCFA) are fatty acids with aliphatic tails of 13 to 21 carbons.

- Very long chain fatty acids (VLCFA) are fatty acids with aliphatic tails of 22 or more carbons.

Any of these aliphatic fatty acid chains may be glycerated and the resultant fats may have tails of different lengths from very short triformin to very long, e.g., cerotic acid, or hexacosanoic acid, a

26-carbon long-chain saturated fatty acid. Long chain fats are exemplified by tallow (lard) whose chains are 17 carbons long. Most fats found in food, whether vegetable or animal, are made up of medium to long-chain fatty acids, usually of equal or nearly equal length. Many cell types can use either glucose or fatty acids for this energy. In particular, heart and skeletal muscle prefer fatty acids. Despite long-standing assertions to the contrary, fatty acids can also be used as a source of fuel for brain cells.

## Importance for Living Organisms

Fats are also sources of essential fatty acids, an important dietary requirement. They provide energy as noted above. Vitamins A, D, E, and K are fat-soluble, meaning they can only be digested, absorbed, and transported in conjunction with fats. Fats play a vital role in maintaining healthy skin and hair, insulating body organs against shock, maintaining body temperature, and promoting healthy cell function. Fat also serves as a useful buffer against a host of diseases. When a particular substance, whether chemical or biotic, reaches unsafe levels in the bloodstream, the body can effectively dilute—or at least maintain equilibrium of—the offending substances by storing it in new fat tissue. This helps to protect vital organs, until such time as the offending substances can be metabolized or removed from the body by such means as excretion, urination, accidental or intentional bloodletting, sebum excretion, and hair growth.

## Adipose Tissue

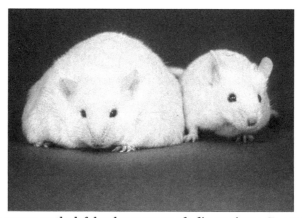

The obese mouse on the left has large stores of adipose tissue. For comparison, a mouse with a normal amount of adipose tissue is shown on the right.

In animals, adipose tissue, or fatty tissue is the body's means of storing metabolic energy over extended periods of time. Adipocytes (fat cells) store fat derived from the diet and from liver metabolism. Under energy stress these cells may degrade their stored fat to supply fatty acids and also glycerol to the circulation. These metabolic activities are regulated by several hormones (e.g., insulin, glucagon and epinephrine). Adipose tissue also secretes the hormone leptin.

The location of the tissue determines its metabolic profile: visceral fat is located within the abdominal wall (i.e., beneath the wall of abdominal muscle) whereas "subcutaneous fat" is located beneath the skin (and includes fat that is located in the abdominal area beneath the skin but *above* the abdominal muscle wall). Visceral fat was recently discovered to be a significant producer of signaling chemicals (i.e., hormones), among which several are involved in inflammatory tissue responses. One of these is resistin which has been linked to obesity, insulin resistance, and Type 2 diabetes. This latter result is currently controversial, and there have been reputable studies supporting all sides on the issue.

## Fatty Acids and Human Health

Dietary consumption of fatty acids has effects on human health. Studies have found that replacing saturated fats with *cis* unsaturated fats in the diet reduces risk of cardiovascular disease. For example, a 2015 systematic review of randomized control trials by the Cochrane Library concluded: "Lifestyle advice to all those at risk of cardiovascular disease and to lower risk population groups should continue to include permanent reduction of dietary saturated fat and partial replacement by unsaturated fats."

Numerous studies have also found that consumption of *trans* fats increases risk of cardiovascular disease. The Harvard School of Public Health advises that replacing *trans* fats and saturated fats with *cis* monounsaturated and polyunsaturated fats is beneficial for health. a 2014 meta-analyses of randomized controlled trials found that reducing fat and cholesterol intake does not affect cardiovascular disease or all-cause mortality.

## Functions of Fat in the Body

Fat is an essential part of your diet. It provides energy, absorbs certain nutrients and maintains your core body temperature. You need to consume fat every day to support these functions, but some types of fat are better for you than others. Good fats protect your heart and keep your body healthy, while bad fats increase your risk of disease and damage your heart.

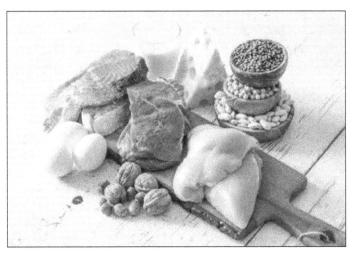

## A Source of Energy

While carbohydrates are the main source of fuel in your body, your system turns to fat as a backup energy source when carbohydrates are not available. Fat is a concentrated source of energy. One gram of fat has 9 calories, which is more than double the amount of calories from carbohydrates and protein. Because fat is high in calories, you need to limit your diet to 20 to 35 percent calories from fat. Based on an 1,800-calorie diet, this recommendation amounts to 40 to 70 daily grams of fat.

## Vitamin Absorption

Some types of vitamins rely on fat for absorption and storage. Vitamins A, D, E and K, called fat-soluble vitamins, cannot function without adequate daily fat intake. These vitamins are essential parts of your daily diet. Vitamin A keeps your eyes healthy and promotes good vision, vitamin D assists in keeping your bones strong by boosting calcium absorption, vitamin E protects cells by neutralizing free radicals and vitamin K is important for blood clotting. If you don't meet your daily fat intake or follow a low-fat diet, absorption of these vitamins may be limited resulting in impaired functioning.

## Insulation and Temperature Regulation

Fat cells, stored in adipose tissue, insulate your body and help sustain a normal core body temperature. Adipose tissue is not always visible, but if you are overweight, you may be able to see it under your skin. You might notice an abundance of adipose tissue in certain areas, causing lumpy patches around your thighs and stomach. Other stored fats surround vital organs and keep them protected from sudden movements or outside impacts.

## Saturated Fat

A saturated fat is a type of fat in which the fatty acid chains have all or predominantly single bonds. A fat is made of two kinds of smaller molecules: glycerol and fatty acids. Fats are made of long chains of carbon (C) atoms. Some carbon atoms are linked by single bonds (-C-C-) and others are linked by double bonds (-C=C-). Double bonds can react with hydrogen to form single bonds. They are called saturated, because the second bond is broken and each half of the bond is attached to (saturated with) a hydrogen atom. Most animal fats are saturated. The fats of plants and fish are generally unsaturated. Saturated fats tend to have higher melting points than their corresponding unsaturated fats, leading to the popular understanding that saturated fats tend to be solids at room temperatures, while unsaturated fats tend to be liquid at room temperature with varying degrees of viscosity (meaning both saturated and unsaturated fats are found to be liquid at body temperature).

Various fats contain different proportions of saturated and unsaturated fat. Examples of foods containing a high proportion of saturated fat include animal fat products such as cream, cheese, butter, other whole milk dairy products and fatty meats which also contain dietary cholesterol. Certain vegetable products have high saturated fat content, such as coconut oil and palm kernel oil. Many prepared foods are high in saturated fat content, such as pizza, dairy desserts, and sausage.

Guidelines released by many medical organizations, including the World Health Organization, have advocated for reduction in the intake of saturated fat to promote health and reduce the risk from cardiovascular diseases. Many articles also recommend a diet low in saturated fat and argue it will lower risks of cardiovascular diseases, diabetes, or death. A small number of contemporary reviews have challenged these conclusions, though predominant medical opinion is that saturated fat and cardiovascular disease are closely related.

## Fat Profiles

While nutrition labels regularly combine them, the saturated fatty acids appear in different proportions among food groups. Lauric and myristic acids are most commonly found in "tropical" oils (e.g., palm kernel, coconut) and dairy products. The saturated fat in meat, eggs, cacao, and nuts is primarily the triglycerides of palmitic and stearic acids.

Table: Saturated fat profile of common foods; esterified fatty acids as percentage of total fat.

| Food | Lauric acid | Myristic acid | Palmitic acid | Stearic acid |
|---|---|---|---|---|
| Coconut oil | 47% | 18% | 9% | 3% |
| Palm kernel oil | 48% | 1% | 44% | 5% |
| Butter | 3% | 11% | 29% | 13% |
| Ground beef | 0% | 4% | 26% | 15% |
| Salmon | 0% | 1% | 29% | 3% |
| Egg yolks | 0% | 0.3% | 27% | 10% |
| Cashews | 2% | 1% | 10% | 7% |
| Soybean oil | 0% | 0% | 11% | 4% |

## Examples of Saturated Fatty Acids

Some common examples of fatty acids:

- Butyric acid with 4 carbon atoms (contained in butter).

- Lauric acid with 12 carbon atoms (contained in coconut oil, palm kernel oil, and breast milk).

- Myristic acid with 14 carbon atoms (contained in cow's milk and dairy products).

- Palmitic acid with 16 carbon atoms (contained in palm oil and meat).

- Stearic acid with 18 carbon atoms (also contained in meat and cocoa butter).

## Dietary Recommendations

Recommendations to reduce or limit dietary intake of saturated fats are made by the World Health Organization, American Heart Association, Health Canada, the US Department of Health and Human Services, the UK National Health Service, the Australian Department of Health and Aging, the Singapore Ministry of Health, the Indian Ministry of Health and Family Wellfare, the New Zealand Ministry of Health, and Hong Kong's Department of Health.

In 2003, the World Health Organization (WHO) and Food and Agriculture Organization (FAO) expert consultation report concluded that "intake of saturated fatty acids is directly related to cardiovascular risk. The traditional target is to restrict the intake of saturated fatty acids to less than 10% of daily energy intake and less than 7% for high-risk groups. If populations are consuming less than 10%, they should not increase that level of intake. Within these limits, intake of foods rich in myristic and palmitic acids should be replaced by fats with a lower content of these particular fatty acids. In developing countries, however, where energy intake for some population groups may be inadequate, energy expenditure is high and body fat stores are low (BMI $<18.5$ kg/m$^2$). The amount and quality of fat supply has to be considered keeping in mind the need to meet energy requirements. Specific sources of saturated fat, such as coconut and palm oil, provide low-cost energy and may be an important source of energy for the poor."

A 2004 statement released by the Centers for Disease Control (CDC) determined that "Americans need to continue working to reduce saturated fat intake." In addition, reviews by the American Heart Association led the Association to recommend reducing saturated fat intake to less than 7% of total calories according to its 2006 recommendations. This concurs with similar conclusions made by the US Department of Health and Human Services, which determined that reduction in saturated fat consumption would positively affect health and reduce the prevalence of heart disease.

The United Kingdom, National Health Service claims the majority of British people eat too much saturated fat. The British Heart Foundation also advises people to cut down on saturated fat. People are advised to cut down on saturated fat and read labels on food they buy.

A 2004 review stated that "no lower safe limit of specific saturated fatty acid intakes has been identified" and recommended that the influence of varying saturated fatty acid intakes against a background of different individual lifestyles and genetic backgrounds should be the focus in future studies.

Blanket recommendations to lower saturated fat were criticized at a 2010 conference debate of the American Dietetic Association for focusing too narrowly on reducing saturated fats rather than emphasizing increased consumption of healthy fats and unrefined carbohydrates. Concern was expressed over the health risks of replacing saturated fats in the diet with refined carbohydrates, which carry a high risk of obesity and heart disease, particularly at the expense of polyunsaturated fats which may have health benefits. None of the panelists recommended heavy consumption of saturated fats, emphasizing instead the importance of overall dietary quality to cardiovascular health.

In a 2017 comprehensive review of the literature and clinical trials, the American Heart Association published a recommendation that saturated fat intake be reduced or replaced by products containing monounsaturated and polyunsaturated fats, a dietary adjustment that could reduce the risk of cardiovascular diseases by 30%.

## Unsaturated Fat

An unsaturated fat is a fat or fatty acid in which there is at least a single double bond within the fatty acid chain. A fatty acid chain is monounsaturated if it contains one double bond, and polyunsaturated if it contains more than one double bond.

Where double bonds are formed, hydrogen atoms are subtracted from the carbon chain. Thus, a saturated fat has no double bonds, has the maximum number of hydrogens bonded to the carbons, and therefore is "saturated" with hydrogen atoms. In cellular metabolism, unsaturated fat molecules contain somewhat less energy (i.e., fewer calories) than an equivalent amount of saturated fat. The greater the degree of unsaturation in a fatty acid (i.e., the more double bonds in the fatty acid) the more vulnerable it is to lipid peroxidation (rancidity). Antioxidants can protect unsaturated fat from lipid peroxidation.

Double bonds may be in either a cis or a trans isomer, depending on the geometry of the double bond. In the cis isomer, hydrogen atoms are on the same side of the double bond; whereas in the trans isomer, they are on opposite sides of the double bond. Saturated fats are useful in processed foods because saturated fats are less vulnerable to rancidity and usually more solid at room temperature than unsaturated fats. Unsaturated chains have a lower melting point, hence these molecules increase the fluidity of cell membranes.

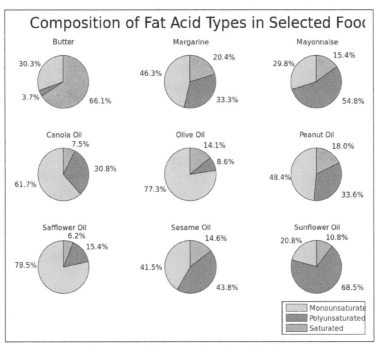

Amounts of fat types in selected foods.

Although both monounsaturated and polyunsaturated fats can replace saturated fat in the diet, trans unsaturated fats should not. Replacing saturated fats with unsaturated fats helps lower levels of total cholesterol and LDL cholesterol in the blood. Trans unsaturated fats are an exception because the double bond stereochemistry predisposes the carbon chains to assume a linear conformation, which conforms to rigid packing as in plaque formation. The geometry of the cis double bond induces a bend in the molecule, thereby precluding rigid formations. Natural sources of fatty acids are rich in the cis isomer.

Although polyunsaturated fats are protective against cardiac arrhythmias, a study of post-menopausal women with a relatively low fat intake showed that polyunsaturated fat is positively associated with progression of coronary atherosclerosis, whereas monounsaturated fat is not. This probably is an indication of the greater vulnerability of polyunsaturated fats to lipid peroxidation, against which vitamin E has been shown to be protective.

Examples of unsaturated fatty acids are palmitoleic acid, oleic acid, myristoleic acid, linoleic acid, and arachidonic acid. Foods containing unsaturated fats include avocado, nuts, olive oils, and vegetable oils such as canola. Meat products contain both saturated and unsaturated fats.

Although unsaturated fats are conventionally regarded as 'healthier' than saturated fats, the United States Food and Drug Administration (FDA) recommendation stated that the amount of unsaturated fat consumed should not exceed 30% of one's daily caloric intake. Most foods contain both unsaturated and saturated fats. Marketers advertise only one or the other, depending on which one makes up the majority. Thus, various unsaturated fat vegetable oils, such as olive oils, also contain saturated fat.

In chemical analysis, fatty acids are separated by gas chromatography of methyl esters; additionally, a separation of unsaturated isomers is possible by argentation thin-layer chromatography.

## Role of Dietary Fats in Insulin Resistance

Incidence of insulin resistance is lowered with diets higher in monounsaturated fats (especially oleic acid), while the opposite is true for diets high in polyunsaturated fats (especially large amounts of arachidonic acid) as well as saturated fats (such as arachidic acid). These ratios can be indexed in the phospholipids of human skeletal muscle and in other tissues as well. This relationship between dietary fats and insulin resistance is presumed secondary to the relationship between insulin resistance and inflammation, which is partially modulated by dietary fat ratios (Omega-3/6/9) with both omega 3 and 9 thought to be anti-inflammatory, and omega 6 pro-inflammatory (as well as by numerous other dietary components, particularly polyphenols and exercise, with both of these anti-inflammatory). Although both pro- and anti-inflammatory types of fat are biologically necessary, fat dietary ratios in most US diets are skewed towards Omega 6, with subsequent disinhibition of inflammation and potentiation of insulin resistance. But this is contrary to the suggestion of more recent studies, in which polyunsaturated fats are shown as protective against insulin resistance.

## Membrane Composition as a Metabolic Pacemaker

Studies on the cell membranes of mammals and reptiles discovered that mammalian cell membranes are composed of a higher proportion of polyunsaturated fatty acids (DHA, omega-3 fatty acid) than reptiles. Studies on bird fatty acid composition have noted similar proportions to mammals but with 1/3rd less omega-3 fatty acids as compared to omega-6 for a given body size. This fatty acid composition results in a more fluid cell membrane but also one that is permeable to various ions (H+ & Na+), resulting in cell membranes that are more costly to maintain. This maintenance cost has been argued to be one of the key causes for the high metabolic rates and concomitant warm-bloodedness of mammals and birds. However polyunsaturation of cell membranes may also occur in response to chronic cold temperatures as well. In fish increasingly cold environments lead to increasingly high cell membrane content of both monounsaturated and polyunsaturated fatty acids, to maintain greater membrane fluidity (and functionality) at the lower temperatures.

## Monounsaturated Fat

In biochemistry and nutrition, monounsaturated fatty acids (abbreviated MUFAs, or more plainly monounsaturated fats) are fatty acids that have one double bond in the fatty acid chain with all of the remainder carbon atoms being single-bonded. By contrast, polyunsaturated fatty acids (PUFAs) have more than one double bond.

## Molecular Description

Fatty acids are long-chained molecules having an alkyl group at one end and a carboxylic acid group at the other end. Fatty acid viscosity (thickness) and melting temperature increases with decreasing number of double bonds; therefore, monounsaturated fatty acids have a higher melting point than polyunsaturated fatty acids (more double bonds) and a lower melting point than saturated fatty acids (no double bonds). Monounsaturated fatty acids are liquids at room temperature and semisolid or solid when refrigerated resulting in a isotopic lattice structure.

Common monounsaturated fatty acids are palmitoleic acid (16:1 n−7), cis-vaccenic acid (18:1 n−7) and oleic acid (18:1 n−9). Palmitoleic acid has 16 carbon atoms with the first double bond occurring

7 carbon atoms away from the methyl group (and 9 carbons from the carboxyl end). It can be lengthened to the 18-carbon cis-vaccenic acid. Oleic acid has 18 carbon atoms with the first double bond occurring 9 carbon atoms away from the carboxylic acid group. The illustrations below show a molecule of oleic acid in Lewis formula and as a space-filling model.

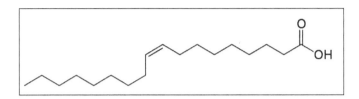 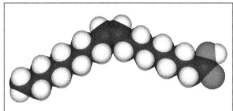

## List of Monounsaturated Fats

| Common name | Lipid name | Chemical name |
|---|---|---|
| Myristoleic acid | 14:1 (n-5) | cis-Tetradec-9-enoic acid |
| Palmitoleic acid | 16:1 (n-7) | cis-Hexadec-9-enoic acid |
| cis-Vaccenic acid | 18:1 (n-7) | cis-Octadec-11-enoic acid |
| Vaccenic acid | 18:1 (n-7) | trans-Octadec-11-enoic acid |
| Paullinic acid | 20:1 (n-7) | cis-13-Eicosenoic acid |
| Oleic acid | 18:1 (n-9) | cis-Octadec-9-enoic acid |
| Elaidic acid (trans-oleic acid) | 18:1 (n-9) | trans-Octadec-9-enoic acid |
| 11-Eicosenoic acid (gondoic acid) | 20:1 (n-9) | cis-Eicos-11-enoic acid |
| Erucic acid | 22:1 (n-9) | cis-Tetracos-15-enoic acid |
| Brassidic acid | 22:1 (n-9) | trans-Tetracos-15-enoic acid |
| Nervonic acid | 24:1 (n-9) | cis-Tetracos-15-enoic acid |
| Sapienic acid | 16:1 (n-10) | cis-6-Hexadecenoic acid |
| Gadoleic acid | 20:1 (n-11) | cis-9-Icosenoic acid |
| Petroselinic acid | 18:1 (n-12) | cis-Octadec-6-enoic acid |

## Health

Monounsaturated fats protect against cardiovascular disease by providing more membrane fluidity than saturated fats, but they are more vulnerable to lipid peroxidation (rancidity). The large scale KANWU study found that increasing monounsaturated fat and decreasing saturated fat intake could improve insulin sensitivity, but only when the overall fat intake of the diet was low. However, some monounsaturated fatty acids (in the same way as saturated fats) may promote insulin resistance, whereas polyunsaturated fatty acids may be protective against insulin resistance. Studies have shown that substituting dietary monounsaturated fat for saturated fat is associated with increased daily physical activity and resting energy expenditure. More physical activity was associated with a higher-oleic acid diet than one of a palmitic acid diet. From the study, it is shown that more monounsaturated fats lead to less anger and irritability.

Foods containing monounsaturated fats reduce low-density lipoprotein (LDL) cholesterol, while possibly increasing high-density lipoprotein (HDL) cholesterol.

Levels of oleic acid along with other monounsaturated fatty acids in red blood cell membranes were positively associated with breast cancer risk. The saturation index (SI) of the same membranes was inversely associated with breast cancer risk. Monounsaturated fats and low SI in erythrocyte membranes are predictors of postmenopausal breast cancer. Both of these variables depend on the activity of the enzyme delta-9 desaturase (Δ9-d).

In children, consumption of monounsaturated oils is associated with healthier serum lipid profiles.

The Mediterranean diet is one heavily influenced by monounsaturated fats. People in Mediterranean countries consume more total fat than Northern European countries, but most of the fat is in the form of monounsaturated fatty acids from olive oil and omega-3 fatty acids from fish, vegetables, and certain meats like lamb, while consumption of saturated fat is minimal in comparison. A 2017 review found evidence that the practice of a Mediterranean diet could lead to a decreased risk of cardiovascular diseases, overall cancer incidence, neurodegenerative diseases, diabetes, and early death. A 2018 review showed that the practice of the Mediterranean diet may improve overall health status, such as reduced risk of non-communicable diseases, reduced total costs of living, and reduced costs for national.

Monounsaturated fats are found in animal flesh such as red meat, whole milk products, nuts, and high fat fruits such as olives and avocados. Olive oil is about 75% monounsaturated fat. The high oleic variety sunflower oil contains as least 70% monounsaturated fat. Canola oil and cashews are both about 58% monounsaturated fat. Tallow (beef fat) is about 50% monounsaturated fat. and lard is about 40% monounsaturated fat. Other sources include avocado oil, macadamia nut oil, grapeseed oil, groundnut oil (peanut oil), sesame oil, corn oil, popcorn, whole grain wheat, cereal, oatmeal, almond oil, sunflower oil, hemp oil, and tea-oil Camellia.

## Polyunsaturated Fat

Polyunsaturated fats are fats in which the constituent hydrocarbon chain possesses two or more carbon–carbon double bonds. Polyunsaturated fat can be found mostly in nuts, seeds, fish, seed oils, and oysters. "Unsaturated" refers to the fact that the molecules contain less than the maximum amount of hydrogen (if there were no double bonds). These materials exist as *cis* or *trans* isomers depending on the geometry of the double bond.

Saturated fats have hydrocarbon chains which can be most readily aligned. The hydrocarbon chains in trans fats align more readily than those in cis fats, but less well than those in saturated fats. In general, this means that the melting points of fats increase from cis to trans unsaturated and then to saturated.

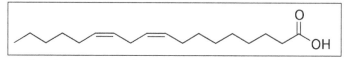

Chemical structure of the polyunsaturated fat linoleic acid.

The position of the carbon-carbon double bonds in carboxylic acid chains in fats is designated by Greek letters. The carbon atom closest to the carboxyl group is the alpha carbon, the next carbon is the beta carbon and so on. In fatty acids the carbon atom of the methyl group at the end of the hydrocarbon chain is called the omega carbon because omega is the last letter of the Greek alphabet.

Omega-3 fatty acids have a double bond three carbons away from the methyl carbon, whereas omega-6 fatty acids have a double bond six carbons away from the methyl carbon. The illustration below shows the omega-6 fatty acid, linoleic acid.

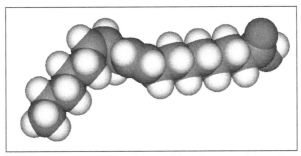

3D representation of linoleic acid in a bent conformation.

While it is the nutritional aspects of polyunsaturated fats that are generally of greatest interest, these materials also have non-food applications. Drying oils, which polymerize on exposure to oxygen to form solid films, are polyunsaturated fats. The most common ones are linseed (flax seed) oil, tung oil, poppy seed oil, perilla oil, and walnut oil. These oils are used to make paints and varnishes.

## Health

## Potential Benefits

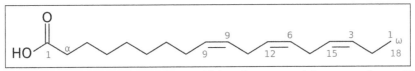

Chemical structure of alpha-linolenic acid (ALA), an essential omega–3 fatty acid.

Because of their effects in the diet, unsaturated fats (monounsaturated and polyunsaturated) are often referred to as *good fats*; while saturated fats are sometimes referred to as *bad fats*. Some fat is needed in the diet, but it is usually considered that fats should not be consumed excessively, unsaturated fats should be preferred, and saturated fats in particular should be limited.

In preliminary research, omega-3 fatty acids in algal oil, fish oil, fish and seafood have been shown to lower the risk of heart attacks. Other preliminary research indicates that omega-6 fatty acids in sunflower oil and safflower oil may also reduce the risk of cardiovascular disease.

Among omega-3 fatty acids, neither long-chain nor short-chain forms were consistently associated with breast cancer risk. High levels of docosahexaenoic acid (DHA), however, the most abundant omega-3 polyunsaturated fatty acid in erythrocyte (red blood cell) membranes, were associated with a reduced risk of breast cancer. The DHA obtained through the consumption of polyunsaturated fatty acids is positively associated with cognitive and behavioral performance. In addition DHA is vital for the grey matter structure of the human brain, as well as retinal stimulation and neurotransmission.

Contrary to conventional advice, an evaluation of evidence from 1966-1973 pertaining to the health impacts of replacing dietary saturated fat with linoleic acid found that participants in the group doing so had *increased* rates of death from all causes, coronary heart disease, and cardiovascular disease. Although this evaluation was disputed by many scientists, it fueled debate over worldwide dietary advice to substitute polyunsaturated fats for saturated fats.

## Pregnancy

Polyunsaturated fat supplementation does not decrease the incidence of pregnancy-related disorders, such as hypertension or preeclampsia, but may increase the length of gestation slightly and decreased the incidence of early premature births.

Expert panels in the United States and Europe recommend that pregnant and lactating women consume higher amounts of polyunsaturated fats than the general population to enhance the DHA status of the fetus and newborn.

## Cancer

Results from observational clinical trials on polyunsaturated fat intake and cancer have been inconsistent and vary by numerous factors of cancer incidence, including gender and genetic risk. Some studies have shown associations between higher intakes and/or blood levels of polyunsaturated fat omega-3s and a decreased risk of certain cancers, including breast and colorectal cancer, while other studies found no associations with cancer risk.

## Food Sources

Food sources of polyunsaturated fats include:

| Food source (100g) | Polyunsaturated fat (g) |
|---|---|
| Walnuts | 47 |
| Canola Oil | 34 |
| Sunflower seeds | 33 |
| Sesame Seeds | 26 |
| Chia Seeds | 23.7 |
| Unsalted Peanuts | 16 |
| Peanut Butter | 14.2 |
| Avocado Oil | 13.5 |
| Olive Oil | 11 |
| Safflower Oil | 12.82 |
| Seaweed | 11 |
| Sardines | 5 |
| Soybeans | 7 |
| Tuna | 14 |
| Wild Salmon | 17.3 |
| Whole Grain Wheat | 9.7 |

## Trans Fat

Trans fat, also called trans-unsaturated fatty acids or trans fatty acids, is a type of unsaturated fat that occurs in small amounts in meat and milk fat. It became widely produced industrially from vegetable and fish oils in the early 20th century for use in margarine and later also in snack food, packaged baked goods, and for frying fast food.

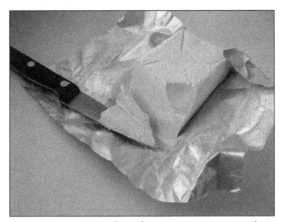
Margarine, a common product that can contain trans fatty acids.

Fats contain long hydrocarbon chains, which can be either unsaturated, i.e., have double bonds, or saturated, i.e., have no double bonds. In nature, unsaturated fatty acids generally have *cis* as opposed to *trans* configurations. In food production, liquid cis-unsaturated fats such as vegetable oils are hydrogenated to produce saturated fats, which have more desirable physical properties: e.g., they melt at a desirable temperature (30–40 °C); and extend the shelf-life of food. Partial hydrogenation of the unsaturated fat converts some of the cis double bonds into trans double bonds by an isomerization reaction with the catalyst used for the hydrogenation, which yields a trans fat.

Although trans fats are edible, consuming trans fats has been shown to increase the risk of coronary artery disease in part by raising levels of low-density lipoprotein (LDL, often termed "bad cholesterol"), lowering levels of high-density lipoprotein (HDL, often termed "good cholesterol"), increasing triglycerides in the bloodstream and promoting systemic inflammation.

Trans fats also occur naturally, e.g., the vaccenic acid in breast milk, and some isomers of conjugated linoleic acid (CLA). These trans fats occur naturally in meat and dairy products from ruminants. Butter, for example, contains about 3% trans fat. Two Canadian studies have shown that vaccenic acid could be beneficial compared to hydrogenated vegetable shortening, or a mixture of pork lard and soy fat, by lowering total LDL and triglyceride levels. A study by the US Department of Agriculture showed that vaccenic acid raises both HDL and LDL cholesterol, whereas industrial trans fats only raise LDL with no beneficial effect on HDL.

In light of recognized evidence and scientific agreement, nutritional authorities consider all trans fats equally harmful for health and recommend that their consumption be reduced to trace amounts. The World Health Organization recommended that trans fats make up no more than 1% of a person's diet in 2003 and, in 2018, introduced a 6-step guide to eliminate industrially-produced trans-fatty acids from the global food supply.

In many countries, there are legal limits to trans fat content. Trans fats levels can be reduced or eliminated by switching to saturated fats such as lard, palm oil, or fully hydrogenated fats, or by using interesterified fat. Other alternative formulations can also allow unsaturated fats to be used to replace saturated or partially hydrogenated fats. Hydrogenated oil is not a synonym for trans fat: complete hydrogenation removes all unsaturated fats.

In chemical terms, trans fat is a fat (lipid) molecule that contains one or more double bonds in trans geometric configuration.

A double bond may exhibit one of two possible configurations: *trans* or *cis*. In *trans* configuration, the carbon chain extends from opposite sides of the double bond, whereas, in *cis* configuration, the carbon chain extends from the same side of the double bond. The *trans* molecule is a straighter molecule. The *cis* molecule is bent.

| Trans (Elaidic acid) | Unsaturated (Oleic acid) | Saturated (Stearic acid) |
|---|---|---|
| Elaidic acid is the main trans unsaturated fatty acid often found in partially hydrogenated vegetable oils. | Oleic acid is an unsaturated fatty acid making up 55–80% of olive oil. | Stearic acid is a saturated fatty acid found in animal fats and is the intended product in full hydrogenation. Stearic acid is neither unsaturated nor trans because it has no carbon-carbon double bonds. |
| | | |
| | | |
| These fatty acids are geometric isomers (structurally identical except for the arrangement of the double bond). | | This fatty acid contains no carbon-carbon double bonds and is not isomeric with the prior two. |

A fatty acid is characterized as either *saturated* or *unsaturated* based on the presence of double bonds in its structure. If the molecule contains no double bonds, it is said to be saturated; otherwise, it is unsaturated to some degree.

Only unsaturated fats can be *trans or cis* fat, since only a double bond can be locked to these orientations. Saturated fatty acids are never called *trans fats* because they have no double bonds. Thus, all their bonds are freely rotatable. Other types of fatty acids, such as crepenynic acid, which contains a triple bond, are rare and of no nutritional significance.

Carbon atoms are tetravalent, forming four covalent bonds with other atoms, whereas hydrogen atoms bond with only one other atom. In saturated fatty acids, each carbon atom (besides the last) is connected to its two neighbour carbon atoms and to two hydrogen atoms. In unsaturated fatty acids, the carbon atoms that are missing a hydrogen atom are joined by double bonds rather than single bonds so that each carbon atom still participates in four bonds.

Hydrogenation of an unsaturated fatty acid refers to the addition of hydrogen atoms to the acid, causing double bonds to become single ones, as carbon atoms acquire new hydrogen partners (to maintain four bonds per carbon atom). Full hydrogenation results in a molecule containing the maximum amount of hydrogen (in other words, the conversion of an unsaturated fatty acid into a saturated one). Partial hydrogenation results in the addition of hydrogen atoms at some of the empty positions, with a corresponding reduction in the number of double bonds. Typical commercial hydrogenation is partial to obtain a malleable mixture of fats that is solid at room temperature, but melts during baking, or consumption.

In most naturally occurring unsaturated fatty acids, the hydrogen atoms are on the same side of the double bonds of the carbon chain. However, partial hydrogenation reconfigures most of the double bonds that do not become chemically saturated, twisting them so that the hydrogen atoms end up on different sides of the chain. This type of configuration is called *trans*, The trans configuration is the lower energy form, and is favored when catalytically equilibrated as a side reaction in hydrogenation.

The same molecule, containing the same number of atoms, with a double bond in the same location, can be either a *trans* or a *cis* fatty acid depending on the configuration of the double bond. For example, oleic acid and elaidic acid are both unsaturated fatty acids with the chemical formula $C_9H_{17}C_9H_{17}O_2$. They both have a double bond located midway along the carbon chain. It is the configuration of this bond that sets them apart. The configuration has implications for the physical-chemical properties of the molecule. The *trans* configuration is straighter, while the *cis* configuration is noticeably kinked as can be seen from the three-dimensional representation shown above.

The *trans* fatty acid elaidic acid has different chemical and physical properties, owing to the slightly different bond configuration. It has a much higher melting point, 45 °C, than oleic acid, 13.4 °C, due to the ability of the trans molecules to pack more tightly, forming a solid that is more difficult to break apart. This notably means that it is a solid at human body temperatures.

In food production, the goal is not to simply change the configuration of double bonds while maintaining the same ratios of hydrogen to carbon. Instead, the goal is to decrease the number of double bonds and increase the amount of hydrogen in the fatty acid. This changes the consistency of the fatty acid and makes it less prone to rancidity (in which free radicals attack double bonds). Production of trans fatty acids is thus an undesirable side effect of partial hydrogenation.

Catalytic partial hydrogenation necessarily produces trans-fats, because of the reaction mechanism. In the first reaction step, one hydrogen is added, with the other, coordinatively unsaturated, carbon being attached to the catalyst. The second step is the addition of hydrogen to the remaining carbon, producing a saturated fatty acid. The first step is reversible, such that the hydrogen is readsorbed on the catalyst and the double bond is re-formed. The intermediate with only one hydrogen added contains no double bond and can freely rotate. Thus, the double bond can re-form as either cis or trans, of which trans is favored, regardless the starting material. Complete hydrogenation also hydrogenates any produced trans fats to give saturated fats.

Researchers at the United States Department of Agriculture have investigated whether hydrogenation can be achieved without the side effect of trans fat production. They varied the pressure under which the chemical reaction was conducted – applying 1400 kPa (200 psi) of pressure to soybean oil in a 2-liter vessel while heating it to between 140 °C and 170 °C. The standard 140 kPa (20 psi) process of hydrogenation produces a product of about 40% trans fatty acid by weight, compared to about 17% using the high-pressure method. Blended with unhydrogenated liquid soybean oil, the high-pressure-processed oil produced margarine containing 5 to 6% trans fat. Based on current U.S. labeling requirements, the manufacturer could claim the product was free of trans fat. The level of trans fat may also be altered by modification of the temperature and the length of time during hydrogenation.

Trans fat levels may be measured. Measurement techniques include chromatography (by silver ion chromatography on thin layer chromatography plates, or small high-performance liquid chromatography columns of silica gel with bonded phenylsulfonic acid groups whose hydrogen atoms have been exchanged for silver ions). The role of silver lies in its ability to form complexes with unsaturated compounds. Gas chromatography and mid-infrared spectroscopy are other methods in use.

## Presence in Food

Table: Trans fat contents in various foods, ranked in g per 100 g.

| Food type | Trans fat content |
|---|---|
| Shortenings | 10g to 33 g |
| Margarine, spreads | 0.2 to 26 g |
| Butter | 2g to 7 g |
| Whole milk | 0.07g to 0.1 g |
| Breads/cake products | 0.1g to 10 g |
| Cookies and crackers | 1g to 8 g |
| Salty snacks | 0g to 4 g |
| Cake frostings, sweets | 0.1g to 7 g |
| Animal fat | 0g to 5 g |
| Ground beef | 1 g |

A type of trans fat occurs naturally in the milk and body fat of ruminants (such as cattle and sheep) at a level of 2–5% of total fat. Natural trans fats, which include conjugated linoleic acid (CLA) and vaccenic acid, originate in the rumen of these animals. CLA has two double bonds, one in the cis configuration and one in trans, which makes it simultaneously a cis- and a trans-fatty acid.

Animal-based fats were once the only *trans* fats consumed, but by far the largest amount of *trans* fat consumed today is created by the processed food industry as a side effect of partially hydrogenating unsaturated plant fats (generally vegetable oils). These partially hydrogenated fats have displaced natural solid fats and liquid oils in many areas, the most notable ones being in the fast food, snack food, fried food, and baked goods industries.

Partially hydrogenated oils have been used in food for many reasons. Hydrogenation increases product shelf life and decreases refrigeration requirements. Many baked foods require semi-solid fats to suspend solids at room temperature; partially hydrogenated oils have the right consistency to replace animal fats such as butter and lard at lower cost. They are also an inexpensive alternative to other semi-solid oils such as palm oil.

Up to 45% of the total fat in those foods containing man-made trans fats formed by partially hydrogenating plant fats may be trans fat. Baking shortenings, unless reformulated, contain around 30% trans fats compared to their total fats. High-fat dairy products such as butter contain about 4%. Margarines not reformulated to reduce trans fats may contain up to 15% trans fat by weight, but some reformulated ones are less than 1% trans fat.

It has been established that *trans* fats in human breast milk fluctuate with maternal consumption of trans fat, and that the amount of trans fats in the bloodstream of breastfed infants fluctuates with the amounts found in their milk. In 1999, reported percentages of trans fats (compared to total fats) in human milk ranged from 1% in Spain, 2% in France, 4% in Germany, and 7% in Canada and the United States.

Reaction scheme.

By far the largest amount of *trans* fat consumed today is created by the processed food industry as a side effect of partially catalytic hydrogenation of unsaturated plant fats (generally vegetable oils) with *cis* carbon-carbon double bonds. These partially hydrogenated fats have displaced natural solid fats and liquid oils in many areas, the most notable ones being in the fast food, snack food, fried food, and baked goods industries.

Trans fats are used in shortenings for deep-frying in restaurants, as they can be used for longer than most conventional oils before becoming rancid. In the early 21st century, non-hydrogenated vegetable oils that have lifespans exceeding that of the frying shortenings became available. As fast-food chains routinely use different fats in different locations, trans fat levels in fast food can have large variations. For example, an analysis of samples of McDonald's French fries collected in 2004 and 2005 found that fries served in New York City contained twice as much trans fat as in Hungary, and 28 times as much as in Denmark, where trans fats are restricted. At KFC, the pattern was reversed, with Hungary's product containing twice the trans fat of the New York product. Even within the United States there was variation, with fries in New York containing 30% more trans fat than those from Atlanta.

## Nutritional Guidelines

The National Academy of Sciences (NAS) advises the United States and Canadian governments on nutritional science for use in public policy and product labeling programs. Their 2002 Dietary Reference Intakes for Energy, Carbohydrate, Fiber, Fat, Fatty Acids, Cholesterol, Protein, and Amino Acids contains their findings and recommendations regarding consumption of trans fat.

Their recommendations are based on two key facts. First, "trans fatty acids are not essential and provide no known benefit to human health", whether of animal or plant origin. Second, while both saturated and trans fats increase levels of LDL, trans fats also lower levels of HDL; thus increasing the risk of coronary artery disease. The NAS is concerned "that dietary trans fatty acids are more deleterious with respect to coronary artery disease than saturated fatty acids". This analysis is supported by a 2006 New England Journal of Medicine (NEJM) scientific review that states "from a nutritional standpoint, the consumption of trans fatty acids results in considerable potential harm but no apparent benefit."

Because of these facts and concerns, the NAS has concluded there is no safe level of trans fat consumption. There is no adequate level, recommended daily amount or tolerable upper limit for trans fats. This is because any incremental increase in trans fat intake increases the risk of coronary artery disease.

Despite this concern, the NAS dietary recommendations have not included eliminating trans fat from the diet. This is because trans fat is naturally present in many animal foods in trace quantities, and thus its removal from ordinary diets might introduce undesirable side effects and nutritional imbalances if proper nutritional planning is not undertaken. The NAS has, thus, "recommended that trans fatty acid consumption be as low as possible while consuming a nutritionally adequate diet". Like the NAS, the World Health Organization has tried to balance public health goals with a practical level of trans fat consumption, recommending in 2003 that trans fats be limited to less than 1% of overall energy intake.

The US National Dairy Council has asserted that the trans fats present in animal foods are of a different type than those in partially hydrogenated oils, and do not appear to exhibit the same negative effects. While a recent scientific review agrees with the conclusion (stating that "the sum of the current evidence suggests that the Public health implications of consuming trans fats from ruminant products are relatively limited"), it cautions that this may be due to the low consumption of trans fats from animal sources compared to artificial ones.

More recent inquiry (independent of the dairy industry) has found in a 2008 Dutch meta-analysis that all trans fats, regardless of natural or artificial origin equally raise LDL and lower HDL levels. Other studies though have shown different results when it comes to animal based trans fats like conjugated linoleic acid (CLA). Although CLA is known for its anticancer properties, researchers have also found that the cis-9, trans-11 form of CLA can reduce the risk for cardiovascular disease and help fight inflammation.

## Health Risks

Partially hydrogenated vegetable oils have been an increasingly significant part of the human diet for about 100 years (in particular, since the later half of the 20th century and where more processed foods are consumed), and some deleterious effects of trans fat consumption are scientifically accepted, forming the basis of the health guidelines.

The exact biochemical process by which trans fats produce specific health problems are a topic of continuing research. Intake of dietary trans fat perturbs the body's ability to metabolize essential fatty acids (EFAs, including Omega-3) leading to changes in the phospholipid fatty acid composition in the aorta, the main artery of the heart, thereby raising risk of coronary artery disease.

While the mechanisms through which trans fatty acids contribute to coronary artery disease are fairly well understood, the mechanism for their effects on diabetes is still under investigation. They may impair the metabolism of long-chain polyunsaturated fatty acids (LCPUFAs), but maternal pregnancy trans fatty acid intake has been inversely associated with LCPUFAs levels in infants at birth thought to underlie the positive association between breastfeeding and intelligence.

High intake of trans fatty acids can lead to many health problems throughout one's life. They are abundant in fast food restaurants. They are consumed in greater quantities by people who lack access to a diet consisting of fewer hydrogenated fats, or who often consume fast food. A diet high in trans fats can contribute to obesity, high blood pressure, and higher risk for heart disease. Trans fat has also been implicated in the development of Type 2 diabetes.

## Coronary Artery Disease

The primary health risk identified for trans fat consumption is an elevated risk of coronary artery disease (CAD). A 1994 study estimated that over 30,000 cardiac deaths per year in the United States are attributable to the consumption of trans fats. By 2006 upper estimates of 100,000 deaths were suggested.

The major evidence for the effect of trans fat on CAD comes from the Nurses' Health Study – a cohort study that has been following 120,000 female nurses since its inception in 1976. In this study, Hu and colleagues analyzed data from 900 coronary events from the study's population during 14 years of followup. He determined that a nurse's CAD risk roughly doubled (relative risk of 1.93, CI: 1.43 to 2.61) for each 2% increase in trans fat calories consumed (instead of carbohydrate calories). By contrast, for each 5% increase in saturated fat calories (instead of carbohydrate calories) there was a 17% increase in risk (relative risk of 1.17, CI: 0.97 to 1.41). "The replacement of saturated fat or trans unsaturated fat by cis (unhydrogenated) unsaturated fats was associated with larger reductions in risk than an isocaloric replacement by carbohydrates." Hu also reports on the benefits of reducing trans fat consumption. Replacing 2% of food energy from trans fat with non-trans unsaturated fats more than halves the risk of CAD (53%). By comparison, replacing a larger 5% of food energy from saturated fat with non-trans unsaturated fats reduces the risk of CAD by 43%.

Another study considered deaths due to CAD, with consumption of trans fats being linked to an increase in mortality, and consumption of polyunsaturated fats being linked to a decrease in mortality.

There are two accepted tests that measure an individual's risk for coronary artery disease, both blood tests. The first considers ratios of two types of cholesterol, the other the amount of a cell-signalling cytokine called C-reactive protein. The ratio test is more accepted, while the cytokine test may be more powerful but is still being studied. The effect of trans fat consumption has been documented on each as follows:

- Cholesterol ratio: This ratio compares the levels of LDL to HDL. Trans fat behaves like saturated fat by raising the level of LDL, but, unlike saturated fat, it has the additional effect of decreasing levels of HDL. The net increase in LDL/HDL ratio with trans fat is approximately double that due to saturated fat. (Higher ratios are worse.) One randomized crossover study published in 2003 comparing the effect of eating a meal on blood lipids of (relatively) cis and trans fat rich meals showed that cholesteryl ester transfer (CET) was 28% higher after the trans meal than after the cis meal and that lipoprotein concentrations were enriched in apolipoprotein(a) after the trans meals.

- C-reactive protein (CRP): A study of over 700 nurses showed that those in the highest quartile of trans fat consumption had blood levels of CRP that were 73% higher than those in the lowest quartile.

## Other Health Risks

There are suggestions that the negative consequences of trans fat consumption go beyond the cardiovascular risk. In general, there is much less scientific consensus asserting that eating trans fat specifically increases the risk of other chronic health problems:

- Alzheimer's Disease: A study published in Archives of Neurology in February 2003 suggested that the intake of both trans fats and saturated fats promote the development of Alzheimer disease, although not confirmed in an animal model. It has been found that trans fats impaired memory and learning in middle-age rats. The trans-fat eating rats' brains had fewer proteins critical to healthy neurological function. Inflammation in and around the hippocampus, the part of the brain responsible for learning and memory. These are the exact types of changes normally seen at the onset of Alzheimer's, but seen after six weeks, even though the rats were still young.

- Cancer: There is no scientific consensus that consuming trans fats significantly increases cancer risks across the board. The American Cancer Society states that a relationship between trans fats and cancer "has not been determined." One study has found a positive connection between trans fat and prostate cancer. However, a larger study found a correlation between trans fats and a significant decrease in high-grade prostate cancer. An increased intake of trans fatty acids may raise the risk of breast cancer by 75%, suggest the results from the French part of the European Prospective Investigation into Cancer and Nutrition.

- Diabetes: There is a growing concern that the risk of type 2 diabetes increases with trans fat consumption. However, consensus has not been reached. For example, one study found that risk is higher for those in the highest quartile of trans fat consumption. Another study has found no diabetes risk once other factors such as total fat intake and BMI were accounted for.

- Obesity: Research indicates that trans fat may increase weight gain and abdominal fat, despite a similar caloric intake. A 6-year experiment revealed that monkeys fed a trans fat diet gained 7.2% of their body weight, as compared to 1.8% for monkeys on a mono-unsaturated fat diet. Although obesity is frequently linked to trans fat in the popular media, this is generally in the context of eating too many calories; there is not a strong scientific consensus connecting trans fat and obesity, although the 6-year experiment did find such a link, concluding that "under controlled feeding conditions, long-term TFA consumption was an independent factor in weight gain. TFAs enhanced intra-abdominal deposition of fat, even in the absence of caloric excess, and were associated with insulin resistance, with evidence that there is impaired post-insulin receptor binding signal transduction."

- Liver dysfunction: Trans fats are metabolized differently by the liver than other fats and interfere with delta 6 desaturase. Delta 6 desaturase is an enzyme involved in converting essential fatty acids to arachidonic acid and prostaglandins, both of which are important to the functioning of cells.

- Infertility in women: One 2007 study found, "Each 2% increase in the intake of energy from trans unsaturated fats, as opposed to that from carbohydrates, was associated with a 73% greater risk of ovulatory infertility".

- Major depressive disorder: Spanish researchers analysed the diets of 12,059 people over six years and found that those who ate the most trans fats had a 48 per cent higher risk of depression than those who did not eat trans fats. One mechanism may be trans-fats' substitution for docosahexaenoic acid (DHA) levels in the orbitofrontal cortex (OFC). Very high intake of trans-fatty acids (43% of total fat) in mice from 2 to 16 months of age was associated with lowered DHA levels in the brain ($p=0.001$). When the brains of 15 major depressive subjects who had committed suicide were examined post-mortem and compared against 27 age-matched controls, the suicidal brains were found to have 16% less (male average) to 32% less (female average) DHA in the OFC. The OFC controls reward, reward expectation, and empathy (all of which are reduced in depressive mood disorders) and regulates the limbic system.

- Behavioral irritability and aggression: a 2012 observational analysis of subjects of an earlier study found a strong relation between dietary trans fat acids and self-reported behavioral aggression and irritability, suggesting but not establishing causality.

- Diminished memory: In a 2015 article, researchers re-analyzing results from the 1999-2005 UCSD Statin Study argue that "greater dietary trans fatty acid consumption is linked to worse word memory in adults during years of high productivity, adults age <45".

- Acne: According to a 2015 study, trans fats are one of several components of Western pattern diets which promote acne, along with carbohydrates with high glycemic load such as refined sugars or refined starches, milk and dairy products, and saturated fats, while omega-3 fatty acids, which reduce acne, are deficient in Western pattern diets.

# Vitamins

A vitamin is an organic molecule (or related set of molecules) that is an essential micronutrient that an organism needs in small quantities for the proper functioning of its metabolism. Essential nutrients cannot be synthesized in the organism, either at all or not in sufficient quantities, and therefore must be obtained through the diet. Vitamin C can be synthesized by some species but not by others; it is not a vitamin in the first instance but is in the second. The term *vitamin* does not include the three other groups of essential nutrients: minerals, essential fatty acids, and essential amino acids. Most vitamins are not single molecules, but groups of related molecules called vitamers. For example, vitamin E consists of four tocopherols and four tocotrienols. The thirteen vitamins required by human metabolism are: vitamin A (as all-*trans*-retinol, all-*trans*-retinyl-esters, as well as all-*trans*-beta-carotene and other provitamin A carotenoids), vitamin $B_1$ (thiamine), vitamin $B_2$ (riboflavin), vitamin $B_3$ (niacin), vitamin $B_5$ (pantothenic acid), vitamin $B_6$ (pyridoxine), vitamin $B_7$ (biotin), vitamin $B_9$ (folic acid or folate), vitamin $B_{12}$ (cobalamins), vitamin C (ascorbic acid), vitamin D (calciferols), vitamin E (tocopherols and tocotrienols), and vitamin K (quinones).

Vitamins have diverse biochemical functions. Vitamin A acts as a regulator of cell and tissue growth and differentiation. Vitamin D provides a hormone-like function, regulating mineral metabolism for bones and other organs. The B complex vitamins function as enzyme cofactors (coenzymes) or the precursors for them. Vitamins C and E function as antioxidants. Both deficient and excess intake of a vitamin can potentially cause clinically significant illness, although excess intake of water-soluble vitamins is less likely to do so.

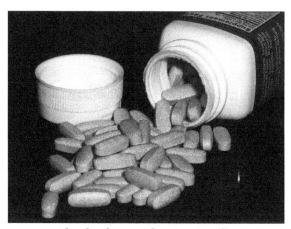

A bottle of B-complex vitamin pills.

Before 1935, the only source of vitamins was from food. If intake of vitamins was lacking, the result was vitamin deficiency and consequent deficiency diseases. Then, commercially produced tablets of yeast-extract vitamin B complex and semi-synthetic vitamin C became available. This was followed in the 1950s by the mass production and marketing of vitamin supplements, including multivitamins, to prevent vitamin deficiencies in the general population. Governments mandated addition of vitamins to staple foods such as flour or milk, referred to as food fortification, to prevent deficiencies. Recommendations for folic acid supplementation during pregnancy reduced risk of infant neural tube defects. Although reducing incidence of vitamin deficiencies clearly has benefits, supplementation is thought to be of little value for healthy people who are consuming a vitamin-adequate diet.

The term *vitamin* is derived from the word *vitamine*, coined in 1912 by Polish biochemist Casimir Funk, who isolated a complex of micronutrients essential to life, all of which he presumed to be amines. When this presumption was later determined not to be true, the "e" was dropped from the name. All vitamins were discovered (identified) between 1913 and 1948.

## Classification

Vitamins are classified as either water-soluble or fat-soluble. In humans there are 13 vitamins: 4 fat-soluble (A, D, E, and K) and 9 water-soluble (8 B vitamins and vitamin C). Water-soluble vitamins dissolve easily in water and, in general, are readily excreted from the body, to the degree that urinary output is a strong predictor of vitamin consumption. Because they are not as readily stored, more consistent intake is important. Fat-soluble vitamins are absorbed through the intestinal tract with the help of lipids (fats). Vitamins A and D can accumulate in the body, which can result in dangerous hypervitaminosis. Fat-soluble vitamin deficiency due to malabsorption is of particular significance in cystic fibrosis.

## Anti-vitamins

Anti-vitamins are chemical compounds that inhibit the absorption or actions of vitamins. For example, avidin is a protein in raw egg whites that inhibits the absorption of biotin; it is deactivated by cooking. Pyrithiamine, a synthetic compound, has a molecular structure similar to thiamine, vitamin $B_1$, and inhibits the enzymes that use thiamine.

## Biochemical Functions

Each vitamin is typically used in multiple reactions, and therefore most have multiple functions.

### On Fetal Growth and Childhood Development

Vitamins are essential for the normal growth and development of a multicellular organism. Using the genetic blueprint inherited from its parents, a fetus develops from the nutrients it absorbs. It requires certain vitamins and minerals to be present at certain times. These nutrients facilitate the chemical reactions that produce among other things, skin, bone, and muscle. If there is serious deficiency in one or more of these nutrients, a child may develop a deficiency disease. Even minor deficiencies may cause permanent damage.

### On Adult Health Maintenance

Once growth and development are completed, vitamins remain essential nutrients for the healthy maintenance of the cells, tissues, and organs that make up a multicellular organism; they also enable a multicellular life form to efficiently use chemical energy provided by food it eats, and to help process the proteins, carbohydrates, and fats required for cellular respiration.

### Intake

For the most part, vitamins are obtained from the diet, but some are acquired by other means: for example, microorganisms in the gut flora produce vitamin K and biotin; and one form of vitamin D is synthesized in skin cells when they are exposed to a certain wavelength of ultraviolet light present in sunlight. Humans can produce some vitamins from precursors they consume: for example, vitamin A is synthesized from beta carotene; and niacin is synthesized from the amino acid tryptophan. The Food Fortification Initiative lists countries which have mandatory fortification programs for vitamins folic acid, niacin, vitamin A and vitamins B1, B2 and B12.

### Deficient Intake

The body's stores for different vitamins vary widely; vitamins A, D, and $B_{12}$ are stored in significant amounts, mainly in the liver, and an adult's diet may be deficient in vitamins A and D for many months and $B_{12}$ in some cases for years, before developing a deficiency condition. However, vitamin $B_3$ (niacin and niacinamide) is not stored in significant amounts, so stores may last only a couple of weeks. For vitamin C, the first symptoms of scurvy in experimental studies of complete vitamin C deprivation in humans have varied widely, from a month to more than six months, depending on previous dietary history that determined body stores.

Deficiencies of vitamins are classified as either primary or secondary. A primary deficiency occurs when an organism does not get enough of the vitamin in its food. A secondary deficiency may be due to an underlying disorder that prevents or limits the absorption or use of the vitamin, due to a "lifestyle factor", such as smoking, excessive alcohol consumption, or the use of medications that interfere with the absorption or use of the vitamin. People who eat a varied diet are unlikely to develop a severe primary vitamin deficiency, but may be consuming less than the recommended amounts; a national food and supplement survey conducted in the US over 2003-2006 reported that over 90% of individuals who did not consume vitamin supplements were found to have inadequate levels of some of the essential vitamins, notably vitamins D and E.

Well-researched human vitamin deficiencies involve thiamine (beriberi), niacin (pellagra), vitamin C (scurvy), folate (neural tube defects) and vitamin D (rickets). In much of the developed world these deficiencies are rare due to an adequate supply of food and the addition of vitamins to common foods. In addition to these classical vitamin deficiency diseases, some evidence has also suggested links between vitamin deficiency and a number of different disorders.

## Excess Intake

Some vitamins have documented acute or chronic toxicity at larger intakes, which is referred to as hypertoxicity. The European Union and the governments of several countries have established Tolerable upper intake levels (ULs) for those vitamins which have documented toxicity. The likelihood of consuming too much of any vitamin from food is remote, but excessive intake (vitamin poisoning) from dietary supplements does occur. In 2016, overdose exposure to all formulations of vitamins and multi-vitamin/mineral formulations was reported by 63,931 individuals to the American Association of Poison Control Centers with 72% of these exposures in children under the age of five. In the US, analysis of a national diet and supplement survey reported that about 7% of adult supplement users exceeded the UL for folate and 5% of those older than age 50 years exceeded the UL for vitamin A.

## Effects of Cooking

The USDA has conducted extensive studies on the percentage losses of various nutrients from different food types and cooking methods. Some vitamins may become more "bio-available" – that is, usable by the body – when foods are cooked. The table below shows whether various vitamins are susceptible to loss from heat—such as heat from boiling, steaming, frying, etc. The effect of cutting vegetables can be seen from exposure to air and light. Water-soluble vitamins such as B and C dissolve into the water when a vegetable is boiled, and are then lost when the water is discarded.

| Vitamin | Soluble in Water | Stable to Air Exposure | Stable to Light Exposure | Stable to Heat Exposure |
|---|---|---|---|---|
| Vitamin A | No | Partially | Partially | Relatively stable |
| Vitamin C | Very unstable | Yes | No | No |
| Vitamin D | No | No | No | No |
| Vitamin E | No | Yes | Yes | No |
| Vitamin K | No | No | Yes | No |
| Thiamine ($B_1$) | Highly | No | ? | > 100 °C |
| Riboflavin ($B_2$) | Slightly | No | In solution | No |

| | | | | |
|---|---|---|---|---|
| Niacin (B$_3$) | Yes | No | No | No |
| Pantothenic acid (b$_5$) | Quite stable | No | No | Yes |
| Vitamin B$_6$ | Yes | ? | Yes | ? |
| Biotin (B$_7$) | Somewhat | ? | ? | No |
| Folic acid (b$_9$) | Yes | ? | When dry | At high temp |
| Cobalamin (B$_{12}$) | Yes | ? | Yes | No |

## Recommended Levels

In setting human nutrient guidelines, government organizations do not necessarily agree on amounts needed to avoid deficiency or maximum amounts to avoid the risk of toxicity. For example, for vitamin C, recommended intakes range from 40 mg/day in India to 155 mg/day for the European Union. The table below shows U.S. Estimated Average Requirements (EARs) and Recommended Dietary Allowances (RDAs) for vitamins, PRIs for the European Union (same concept as RDAs), followed by what three government organizations deem to be the safe upper intake. RDAs are set higher than EARs to cover people with higher than average needs. Adequate Intakes (AIs) are set when there is not sufficient information to establish EARs and RDAs. Governments are slow to revise information of this nature. For the U.S. values, with the exception of calcium and vitamin D, all of the data date to 1997-2004.

| Nutrient | U.S. EAR | Highest U.S. RDA or AI | Highest EU PRI or AI | Upper limit (UL) | | | Unit |
|---|---|---|---|---|---|---|---|
| | | | | U.S. | EU | Japan | |
| Vitamin A | 625 | 900 | 1300 | 3000 | 3000 | 2700 | µg |
| Vitamin C | 75 | 90 | 155 | 2000 | ND | ND | mg |
| Vitamin D | 10 | 15 | 15 | 100 | 100 | 100 | µg |
| Vitamin K | NE | 120 | 70 | ND | ND | ND | µg |
| α-tocopherol (Vitamin E) | 12 | 15 | 13 | 1000 | 300 | 650-900 | mg |
| Thiamin (Vitamin B$_1$) | 1.0 | 1.2 | 0.1 mg/MJ | ND | ND | ND | mg |
| Riboflavin (Vitamin B$_2$) | 1.1 | 1.3 | 2.0 | ND | ND | ND | mg |
| Niacin (Vitamin B$_3$) | 12 | 16 | 1.6 mg/MJ | 35 | 10 | 60-85 | mg |
| Pantothenic acid (Vitamin B$_5$) | NE | 5 | 7 | ND | ND | ND | mg |
| Vitamin B$_6$ | 1.1 | 1.3 | 1.8 | 100 | 25 | 40-60 | mg |
| Biotin (Vitamin B$_7$) | NE | 30 | 45 | ND | ND | ND | µg |
| Folate (Vitamin B$_9$) | 320 | 400 | 600 | 1000 | 1000 | 900-1000 | µg |
| Cyanocobalamin (Vitamin B$_{12}$) | 2.0 | 2.4 | 5.0 | ND | ND | ND | µg |

## Supplementation

In those who are otherwise healthy, there is little evidence that supplements have any benefits with respect to cancer or heart disease. Vitamin A and E supplements not only provide no health benefits for generally healthy individuals, but they may increase mortality, though the two large studies that support this conclusion included smokers for whom it was already known that beta-carotene supplements can be harmful. A 2018 meta-analysis found no evidence that intake of vitamin D or calcium for community-dwelling elderly people reduced bone fractures.

In Europe are regulations that define limits of vitamin (and mineral) dosages for their safe use as dietary supplements. Most vitamins that are sold as dietary supplements are not supposed to exceed a maximum daily dosage referred to as the tolerable upper intake level (UL or Upper Limit). Vitamin products above these regulatory limits are not considered supplements and should be registered as prescription or non-prescription (over-the-counter drugs) due to their potential side effects. The European Union, United States and Japan establish ULs.

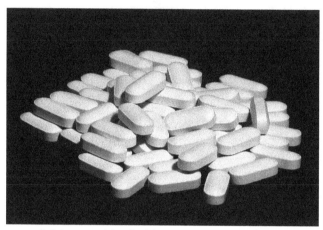

Calcium combined with vitamin D (as calciferol)
supplement tablets with fillers.

Dietary supplements often contain vitamins, but may also include other ingredients, such as minerals, herbs, and botanicals. Scientific evidence supports the benefits of dietary supplements for persons with certain health conditions. In some cases, vitamin supplements may have unwanted effects, especially if taken before surgery, with other dietary supplements or medicines, or if the person taking them has certain health conditions. They may also contain levels of vitamins many times higher, and in different forms, than one may ingest through food.

## Governmental Regulation

Most countries place dietary supplements in a special category under the general umbrella of *foods*, not drugs. As a result, the manufacturer, and not the government, has the responsibility of ensuring that its dietary supplement products are safe before they are marketed. Regulation of supplements varies widely by country. In the United States, a dietary supplement is defined under the Dietary Supplement Health and Education Act of 1994. There is no FDA approval process for dietary supplements, and no requirement that manufacturers prove the safety or efficacy of supplements introduced before 1994. The Food and Drug Administration must rely on its Adverse Event Reporting System to monitor adverse events that occur with supplements. In 2007, the US Code of Federal Regulations (CFR) Title 21, part III took effect, regulating Good Manufacturing Practices (GMPs) in the manufacturing, packaging, labeling, or holding operations for dietary supplements. Even though product registration is not required, these regulations mandate production and quality control standards (including testing for identity, purity and adulterations) for dietary supplements. In the European Union, the Food Supplements Directive requires that only those supplements that have been proven safe can be sold without a prescription. For most vitamins, pharmacopoeial standards have been established. In the United States, the United States Pharmacopeia (USP) sets standards for the most commonly used vitamins and preparations thereof.

Likewise, monographs of the European Pharmacopoeia (Ph.Eur.) regulate aspects of identity and purity for vitamins on the European market.

## Naming

Table: Nomenclature of reclassified vitamins.

| Previous name | Chemical name | Reason for name change |
|---|---|---|
| Vitamin $B_4$ | Adenine | DNA metabolite; synthesized in body. |
| Vitamin $B_8$ | Adenylic acid | DNA metabolite; synthesized in body. |
| Vitamin $B_T$ | Carnitine | Synthesized in body. |
| Vitamin F | Essential fatty acids | Needed in large quantities (does not fit the definition of a vitamin). |
| Vitamin G | Riboflavin | Reclassified as Vitamin $B_2$. |
| Vitamin H | Biotin | Reclassified as Vitamin $B_7$. |
| Vitamin J | Catechol, Flavin | Catechol nonessential; flavin reclassified as Vitamin $B_2$ |
| Vitamin $L_1$ | Anthranilic acid | Non-essential. |
| Vitamin $L_2$ | Adenylthiomethylpentose | RNA metabolite; synthesized in body. |
| Vitamin M | Folic acid | Reclassified as Vitamin $B_9$. |
| Vitamin P | Flavonoids | No longer classified as a vitamin. |
| Vitamin PP | Niacin | Reclassified as Vitamin $B_3$. |
| Vitamin S | Salicylic acid | Proposed inclusion of salicylate as an essential micronutrient. |
| Vitamin U | S-Methylmethionine | Protein metabolite; synthesized in body. |

The reason that the set of vitamins skips directly from E to K is that the vitamins corresponding to letters F–J were either reclassified over time, discarded as false leads, or renamed because of their relationship to vitamin B, which became a complex of vitamins.

The German-speaking scientists who isolated and described vitamin K (in addition to naming it as such) did so because the vitamin is intimately involved in the coagulation of blood following wounding. At the time, most (but not all) of the letters from F through to J were already designated, so the use of the letter K was considered quite reasonable. The table *Nomenclature of reclassified vitamins* lists chemicals that had previously been classified as vitamins, as well as the earlier names of vitamins that later became part of the B-complex.

The missing B vitamins were reclassified or determined not to be vitamins. For example, $B_9$ is folic acid and five of the folates are in the range $B_{11}$ through $B_{16}$. Others, such as PABA (formerly $B_{10}$), are biologically inactive, toxic, or with unclassifiable effects in humans, or not generally recognised as vitamins by science, such as the highest-numbered, which some naturopath practitioners call $B_{21}$ and $B_{22}$. There are also nine lettered B complex vitamins (e.g., $B_m$). There are other D vitamins now recognised as other substances, which some sources of the same type number up to $D_7$. The controversial cancer treatment laetrile was at one point lettered as vitamin $B_{17}$. There appears to be no consensus on any vitamins Q, R, T, V, W, X, Y or Z, nor are there substances officially designated as vitamins N or I, although the latter may have been another form of one of the other vitamins or a known and named nutrient of another type.

# Minerals

Just like vitamins, minerals help your body grow, develop, and stay healthy. The body uses minerals to perform many different functions — from building strong bones to transmitting nerve impulses. Some minerals are even used to make hormones or maintain a normal heartbeat.

## Macro and Trace

The two kinds of minerals are: macrominerals and trace minerals. Macro means "large" (and your body needs larger amounts of macrominerals than trace minerals). The macromineral group is made up of calcium, phosphorus, magnesium, sodium, potassium, chloride, and sulfur.

A trace of something means that there is only a little of it. So even though your body needs trace minerals, it needs just a tiny bit of each one. Trace minerals includes iron, manganese, copper, iodine, zinc, cobalt, fluoride, and selenium.

## Calcium

Calcium is the top macromineral when it comes to your bones. This mineral helps build strong bones, so you can do everything from standing up straight to scoring that winning goal. It also helps build strong, healthy teeth, for chomping on tasty food.

Foods rich in calcium:

- Dairy products, such as milk, cheese, and yogurt.
- Canned salmon and sardines with bones.
- Leafy green vegetables, such as broccoli.
- Calcium-fortified foods — from orange juice to cereals and crackers.

## Iron

The body needs iron to transport oxygen from your lungs to the rest of your body. Your entire body needs oxygen to stay healthy and alive. Iron helps because it's important in the formation of haemoglobin, which is the part of your red blood cells that carries oxygen throughout the body.

Foods rich in iron:

- Meat, especially red meat, such as beef,
- Tuna and salmon,
- Eggs,
- Beans,
- Baked potato with skins,
- Dried fruits, like raisins,

- Leafy green vegetables, such as broccoli,

- Whole and enriched grains, like wheat or oats.

## Potassium

Potassium keeps your muscles and nervous system working properly.

Foods rich in potassium:

- Bananas,

- Tomatoes,

- Potatoes and sweet potatoes, with skins,

- Green vegetables, such as spinach and broccoli,

- Citrus fruits, like oranges,

- Low-fat milk and yogurt,

- Legumes, such as beans, split peas, and lentils.

## Zinc

Zinc helps your immune system, which is your body's system for fighting off illnesses and infections. It also helps with cell growth and helps heal wounds, such as cuts.

Foods rich in zinc:

- Beef, pork, and dark meat chicken,

- Nuts, such as cashews, almonds, and peanuts,

- Legumes, such as beans, split peas, and lentils.

When people don't get enough of these important minerals, they can have health problems. For instance, too little calcium can lead to weaker bones.

## References

- Carbohydrates- 51976: livescience.com, Retrieved 18 June, 2019

- Three-functions-fat-body-3402: healthyeating.sfgate.com, Retrieved 05 May, 2019

- Minerals, kids: kidshealth.org, Retrieved 14 March, 2019

- Gropper SS, Smith JL, Groff JL (2009). Advanced nutrition and human metabolism. Belmont, CA: Wadsworth Cengage Learning. ISBN 978-0-495-11657-8

- Aizpurua-Olaizola O, Ormazabal M, Vallejo A, Olivares M, Navarro P, Etxebarria N, et al. (January 2015). "Optimization of supercritical fluid consecutive extractions of fatty acids and polyphenols from Vitis vinifera grape wastes". Journal of Food Science. 80 (1): E101–7. doi:10.1111/1750-3841.12715. PMID 25471637

# 4

# Common Food Additives

Food additive refers to a chemical substance which is added to food in order to enhance the taste, appearance and preserve its flavor. Anticaking agents, food coloring and glazing agents are a few examples of commonly used food additives. The diverse applications of these additives have been thoroughly discussed in this chapter.

Food additive is any of various chemical substances added to foods to produce specific desirable effects. Additives such as salt, spices, and sulfites have been used since ancient times to preserve foods and make them more palatable. With the increased processing of foods in the 20th century, there came a need for both the greater use of and new types of food additives. Many modern products, such as low-calorie, snack, and ready-to-eat convenience foods, would not be possible without food additives.

There are four general categories of food additives: nutritional additives, processing agents, preservatives, and sensory agents. These are not strict classifications, as many additives fall into more than one category.

## Nutritional Additives

Nutritional additives are used for the purpose of restoring nutrients lost or degraded during production, fortifying or enriching certain foods in order to correct dietary deficiencies, or adding nutrients to food substitutes. The fortification of foods began in 1924 when iodine was added to table salt for the prevention of goitre. Vitamins are commonly added to many foods in order to enrich their nutritional value. For example, vitamins A and D are added to dairy and cereal products, several of the B vitamins are added to flour, cereals, baked goods, and pasta, and vitamin C is added to fruit beverages, cereals, dairy products, and confectioneries. Other nutritional additives include the essential fatty acid linoleic acid, minerals such as calcium and iron, and dietary fibre.

## Processing Agents

A number of agents are added to foods in order to aid in processing or to maintain the desired consistency of the product.

Table: Processing additives and their uses.

| Function | Typical chemical agent | Typical product |
|---|---|---|
| Anticaking | Sodium aluminosilicate | Salt |

| Bleaching | Benzoyl peroxide | Flour |
|---|---|---|
| Chelating | Ethylenediaminetetraacetic acid (edta) | Dressings, mayonnaise, sauces, dried bananas |
| Clarifying | Bentonite, proteins | Fruit juices, wines |
| Conditioning | Potassium bromate | Flour |
| Emulsifying | Lecithin | Ice cream, mayonnaise, bakery products |
| Leavening | Yeast, baking powder, baking soda | Bakery products |
| Moisture control (humectants) | Glycerol | Marshmallows, soft candies, chewing gum |
| Ph control | Citric acid, lactic acid | Certain cheeses, confections, jams and jellies |
| Stabilizing and thickening | Pectin, gelatin, carrageenan, gums (arabic, guar, locust bean) | Dressings, frozen desserts, confections, pudding mixes, jams and jellies |

Emulsifiers are used to maintain a uniform dispersion of one liquid in another, such as oil in water. The basic structure of an emulsifying agent includes a hydrophobic portion, usually a long-chain fatty acid, and a hydrophilic portion that may be either charged or uncharged. The hydrophobic portion of the emulsifier dissolves in the oil phase, and the hydrophilic portion dissolves in the aqueous phase, forming a dispersion of small oil droplets. Emulsifiers thus form and stabilize oil-in-water emulsions (e.g., mayonnaise), uniformly disperse oil-soluble flavor compounds throughout a product, prevent large ice crystal formation in frozen products (e.g., ice cream), and improve the volume, uniformity, and fineness of baked products.

Stabilizers and thickeners have many functions in foods. Most stabilizing and thickening agents are polysaccharides, such as starches or gums, or proteins, such as gelatin. The primary function of these compounds is to act as thickening or gelling agents that increase the viscosity of the final product. These agents stabilize emulsions, either by adsorbing to the outer surface of oil droplets or by increasing the viscosity of the water phase. Thus, they prevent the coalescence of the oil droplets, promoting the separation of the oil phase from the aqueous phase (i.e., creaming). The formation and stabilization of foam in a food product occurs by a similar mechanism, except that the oil phase is replaced by a gas phase. The compounds also act to inhibit the formation of ice or sugar crystals in foods and can be used to encapsulate flavor compounds.

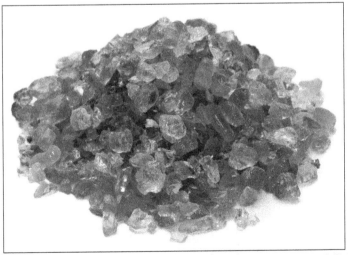

Gum Arabic: Gum arabic from Acacia species. Gum is used as a stabilizing or thickening agent in food to increase the viscosity of the final product.

Chelating, or sequestering, agents protect food products from many enzymatic reactions that promote deterioration during processing and storage. These agents bind to many of the minerals that are present in food (e.g., calcium and magnesium) and are required as cofactors for the activity of certain enzymes.

## Preservatives

Food preservatives are classified into two main groups: antioxidants and antimicrobials. Antioxidants are compounds that delay or prevent the deterioration of foods by oxidative mechanisms. Antimicrobial agents inhibit the growth of spoilage and pathogenic microorganisms in food.

## Antioxidants

The oxidation of food products involves the addition of an oxygen atom to or the removal of a hydrogen atom from the different chemical molecules found in food. Two principal types of oxidation that contribute to food deterioration are autoxidation of unsaturated fatty acids (i.e., those containing one or more double bonds between the carbon atoms of the hydrocarbon chain) and enzyme-catalyzed oxidation.

The autoxidation of unsaturated fatty acids involves a reaction between the carbon-carbon double bonds and molecular oxygen ($O_2$). The products of autoxidation, called free radicals, are highly reactive, producing compounds that cause the off-flavors and off-odours characteristic of oxidative rancidity. Antioxidants that react with the free radicals (called free radical scavengers) can slow the rate of autoxidation. These antioxidants include the naturally occurring tocopherols (vitamin E derivatives) and the synthetic compounds butylated hydroxyanisole (BHA), butylated hydroxytoluene (BHT), and tertiary butylhydroquinone (TBHQ).

Specific enzymes may also carry out the oxidation of many food molecules. The products of these oxidation reactions may lead to quality changes in the food. For example, enzymes called phenolases catalyze the oxidation of certain molecules (e.g., the amino acid tyrosine) hen fruits and vegetables, such as apples, bananas, and potatoes, are cut or bruised. The product of these oxidation reactions, collectively known as enzymatic browning, is a dark pigment called melanin. Antioxidants that inhibit enzyme-catalyzed oxidation include agents that bind free oxygen (i.e., reducing agents), such as ascorbic acid (vitamin C), and agents that inactivate the enzymes, such as citric acid and sulfites.

## Antimicrobials

Antimicrobials are most often used with other preservation techniques, such as refrigeration, in order to inhibit the growth of spoilage and pathogenic microorganisms. Sodium chloride (NaCl), or common salt, is probably the oldest known antimicrobial agent. Organic acids, including acetic, benzoic, propionic, and sorbic acids, are used against microorganisms in products with a low pH. Nitrates and nitrites are used to inhibit the bacterium Clostridium botulinum in cured meat products (e.g., ham and bacon). Sulfur dioxide and sulfites are used to control the growth of spoilage microorganisms in dried fruits, fruit juices, and wines. Nisin and natamycin are preservatives produced by microorganisms. Nisin inhibits the growth of some bacteria, while natamycin is active against molds and yeasts.

## Sensory Agents

## Colorants

Color is an extremely important sensory characteristic of foods; it directly influences the perception of both the flavor and quality of a product. The processing of food can cause degradation or loss of natural pigments in the raw materials. In addition, some formulated products, such as soft drinks, confections, ice cream, and snack foods, require the addition of coloring agents. Colorants are often necessary to produce a uniform product from raw materials that vary in color intensity. Colorants used as food additives are classified as natural or synthetic. Natural colorants are derived from plant, animal, and mineral sources, while synthetic colorants are primarily petroleum-based chemical compounds.

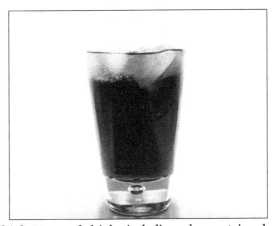

Soft drink: Many soft drinks, including colas, contain colorants.

## Natural Colorants

Most natural colorants are extracts derived from plant tissues. The use of these extracts in the food industry has certain problems associated with it, including the lack of consistent color intensities, instability upon exposure to light and heat, variability of supply, reactivity with other food components, and addition of secondary flavors and odours. In addition, many are insoluble in water and therefore must be added with an emulsifier in order to achieve an even distribution throughout the food product.

Table: Natural food colorants.

| Chemical class | Color | Plant source | Pigment | Products |
|---|---|---|---|---|
| Anthocyanins | Red | Strawberry (fragaria species) | Pelargonidin 3-glucoside | Beverages, confections, preserves, fruit products |
| | Blue | Grape (Vitis species) | Malvidin 3-glucoside | Beverages |
| Betacyanins | Red | Beetroot (beta vulgaris) | Betanin | Dairy products, desserts, icings |
| Carotenoids | Yellow/orange | Annatto (bixa orellana) | Bixin | Dairy products, margarine |
| | Yellow | Saffron (Crocus sativus) | Crocin | Rice dishes, bakery products |
| | Red/orange | Paprika (Capsicum annuum) | Capsanthin | Soups, sauces |
| | Orange | Carrot (Daucus carota) | Beta-carotene | Bakery products, confections |
| | Red | Mushroom (Cantharellus cinnabarinus) | Canthaxanthin | Sauces, soups, dressings |
| Phenolics | Orange/yellow | Turmeric (cuycuma longa) | Curcumin | Dairy products, confections |

## Synthetic Colorants

Synthetic colorants are water-soluble and are available commercially as powders, pastes, granules, or solutions. Special preparations called lakes are formulated by treating the colorants with aluminum hydroxide. They contain approximately 10 to 40 percent of the synthetic dye and are insoluble in water and organic solvents. Lakes are ideal for use in dry and oil-based products. The stability of synthetic colorants is affected by light, heat, pH, and reducing agents. A number of dyes have been chemically synthesized and approved for usage in various countries. These colorants are designated according to special numbering systems specific to individual countries. For example, the United States uses FD&C numbers (chemicals approved for use in foods, drugs, and cosmetics), and the European Union (EU) uses E numbers.

Table: Synthetic food colorants.

| Common name | Designation | | Products |
| | United states | European union | |
|---|---|---|---|
| Allura red AC | FD&C red no. 40 | ... | Gelatin, puddings, dairy products, confections, beverages. |
| Brilliant blue FCF | FD&C blue no. 1 | E133 | Beverages, confections, icings, syrups, dairy products. |
| Erythrosine | Fd&c red no. 3 | E127 | Maraschino cherries. |
| Fast green FCF | FD&C green no. 3 | ... | Beverages, puddings, ice cream, sherbet, confections. |
| Indigo carmine | Fd&c blue no. 2 | E132 | Confections, ice cream, bakery products. |
| Sunset yellow FCF | FD&C yellow no. 6 | E110 | Bakery products, ice cream, sauces, cereals, beverages. |
| Tartrazine | Fd&c yellow no. 5 | E102 | Beverages, cereals, bakery products, ice cream, sauces. |

All synthetic colorants have undergone extensive toxicological analysis. Brilliant Blue FCF, Indigo Carmine, Fast Green FCF, and Erythrosine are poorly absorbed and show little toxicity. Extremely high concentrations (greater than 10 percent) of Allura Red AC cause psychotoxicity, and Tartrazine induces hypersensitive reactions in some persons. Synthetic colorants are not universally approved in all countries.

## Flavorings

The flavor of food results from the stimulation of the chemical senses of taste and smell by specific food molecules. Taste reception is carried out in specialized cells located in the taste buds. The five basic taste sensations—sweet, salty, bitter, sour, and umami—are detected in regions of the tongue, mouth, and throat. Taste cells are specific for certain flavor molecules (e.g., sweeteners).

In addition to the basic tastes, the flavoring molecules in food stimulate specific olfactory (smell) cells in the nasal cavity. These cells can detect more than 10,000 different stimuli, thus fine-tuning the flavor sensation of a food.

A flavor additive is a single chemical or blend of chemicals of natural or synthetic origin that provides all or part of the flavor impact of a particular food. These chemicals are added in order to replace flavor lost in processing and to develop new products. Flavorings are the largest group of food additives, with more than 1,200 compounds available for commercial use. Natural flavorings are derived or extracted from plants, spices, herbs, animals, or microbial fermentations. Artificial flavorings are mixtures of synthetic compounds that may be chemically identical to natural flavorings. Artificial flavorings are often used in food products because of the high cost, lack of availability, or insufficient potency of natural flavorings.

Flavor enhancers are compounds that are added to a food in order to supplement or enhance its own natural flavor. The concept of flavor enhancement originated in Asia, where cooks added seaweed to soup stocks in order to provide a richer flavor to certain foods. The flavor-enhancing component of seaweed was identified as the amino acid L-glutamate, and monosodium glutamate (MSG) became the first flavor enhancer to be used commercially. The rich flavor associated with L-glutamate was called umami.

Other compounds that are used as flavor enhancers include the 5'-ribonucleotides, inosine monophosphate (IMP), guanosine monophosphate (GMP), yeast extract, and hydrolyzed vegetable protein. Flavor enhancers may be used in soups, broths, sauces, gravies, flavoring and spice blends, canned and frozen vegetables, and meats.

## Sweeteners

Sucrose, or table sugar, is the standard on which the relative sweetness of all other sweeteners is based. Because sucrose provides energy in the form of carbohydrates, it is considered a nutritive sweetener. Other nutritive sweeteners include glucose, fructose, corn syrup, high-fructose corn syrup, and sugar alcohols (e.g., sorbitol, mannitol, and xylitol).

Efforts to chemically synthesize sweeteners began in the late 1800s with the discovery of saccharin. Since then, a number of synthetic compounds have been developed that provide few or no calories or nutrients in the diet and are called nonnutritive sweeteners. These sweeteners have significantly greater sweetening power than sucrose, and therefore a relatively low concentration may be used in food products. In addition to saccharin, the most commonly used nonnutritive sweeteners are cyclamates, aspartame, and acesulfame K.

The sensation of sweetness is transmitted through specific protein molecules, called receptors, located on the surface of specialized taste cells. All sweeteners function by binding to these receptors on the outside of the cells. The increased sweetness of the nonnutritive sweeteners relative to sucrose may be due to either tighter or longer binding of these synthetic compounds to the receptors.

Nonnutritive sweeteners are primarily used for the production of low-calorie products including baked goods, confectioneries, dairy products, desserts, preserves, soft drinks, and tabletop sweeteners. They are also used as a carbohydrate replacement for persons with diabetes mellitus and in chewing gum and candies to minimize the risk of dental caries (i.e., tooth decay). Unlike nutritive sweeteners, nonnutritive sweeteners do not provide viscosity or texture to products, so bulking agents such as polydextrose are often required for manufacture.

## Toxicological Testing and Health Concerns

Food additives and their metabolites are subjected to rigorous toxicological analysis prior to their approval for use in the industry. Feeding studies are carried out using animal species (e.g., rats, mice, dogs) in order to determine the possible acute, short-term, and long-term toxic effects of these chemicals. These studies monitor the effects of the compounds on the behaviour, growth, mortality, blood chemistry, organs, reproduction, offspring, and tumour development in the test animals over a 90-day to two-year period. The lowest level of additive producing no toxicological effects is called the no-effect level (NOEL). The NOEL is generally divided by 100 to determine a maximum acceptable daily intake (ADI).

Toxicological analysis of the nonnutritive sweeteners has produced variable results. High concentrations of saccharin and cyclamates in the diets of rats have been shown to induce the development of bladder tumours in the animals. Because of these results, the use of cyclamates has been banned in several countries, including the United States, and the use of saccharin must include a qualifying statement regarding its potential health risks. However, no evidence of human bladder cancer has been reported with the consumption of these sweeteners. Both aspartame and acesulfame K have been deemed to be relatively safe, with no evidence of carcinogenic potential in animal studies.

# Anti Caking Agents

Anticaking agents are food additives that keep powders or granulated materials such as milk powder, powdered sugar, tea and coffee powders used in vending machines, table salt etc. flowing freely. Anti caking agents, in fact, prevent the formation of lumps making these products manageable for packaging, transport and for use by end consumer.

Anticaking agent is the food additive that prevents agglomeration in certain solids, permitting a free-flowing condition. Anticaking agents consist of such substances as starch, magnesium carbonate, and silica and are added to fine-particle solids, such as food products like table salt, flours, coffee, and sugar.

## Examples of Anti Caking Agents in Food

Some of the common examples of foods that contain anti caking agents include:

- Vending machine powders (coffee, cocoa, soup),
- Milk and cream powders,
- Grated cheese,
- Icing sugar,
- Baking powder,
- Cake mixes,
- Instant soup powders,

- Drinking chocolate,

- Table salt.

Anti caking agents are also one of the most common flour treatment agents.

## Functions of Anti Caking Agents

Anticaking agents function either by adsorbing excess moisture, or by coating particles and making them water repellent. Some anticaking agents are soluble in water; others are soluble in alcohols or other organic solvents. Calcium silicate ($CaSiO_3$), a common anti caking agent which is added to table salt etc. adsorbs both water and oil. Although they are food additives, anti caking agents have other applications too. For example, anticaking agents are popularly used in non-food items like road salt, fertilizers, cosmetics, synthetic detergents, and in other such manufacturing applications.

## Manufactured and Natural Anti Caking Agents

There are two types of anti caking agents – manufactured or man-made and natural anticaking agents. Most of the anti caking agents are made from synthetic substances such as silicon dioxide or magnesium and calcium stearates (solid saturated fatty acids.) However, there are many ani caking agents that come from natural sources. Some of the natural anticaking agents include kaolin (E559; talc (E553b); and bentonite. Some anti caking agents manufacturers also produce organic and hypoallergenic anticaking agents from such natural source as rice.

Manmade anticaking agents are manufactured from chemicals and other artificial substances like silicates, acids etc. Examples of manufactured anti caking agents include calcium silicate (E552), magnesium carbonate (E504) and sodium aluminosilicate (E554) etc. Majority of anti caking agents are found with E numbers from 500 to 599. However, apart from the list of E numbers anticaking agents, there are a few that fall into other categories too like the acidity regulators (because they serve two purposes.) Some of such anticaking agents having dual/ multiple purposes include:

E421 - Mannitol as it is also a texturising agent, a sweetening agent, and anti-sticking agent as well as a humectant.

E460a - Microcrystalline cellulose as is also a bulking agent, binder and stabiliser.

E460b - Alpha cellulose as it is also a bulking agent, binder and stabiliser.

## List of Anti Caking Agents E numbers

Table: List of anti caking agents commonly used in foods and drinks.

| E341 - Tricalcium Phosphate | E521 - Aluminium sodium sulphate | E553(a) - (i) Magnesium silicate and (ii) magnesium trisilicate |
|---|---|---|
| E500 - Sodium carbonate | E522 - Aluminium potassium sulphate | E553(b) – Talc |
| E501 - Potassium carbonate | E523 - Aluminium ammonium sulphate | E554 - Sodium aluminium silicate |
| E503 - Ammonium carbonate | E524 - Sodium hydroxide | E555 - Potassium aluminium silicate (Produced from several natural minerals.) |

| | | |
|---|---|---|
| E504 - Magnesium carbonate | E525 - Potassium hydroxide | E556 - Aluminium calcium silicate (Produced from several natural minerals.) |
| E507 - Hydrochloric acid | E526 - Calcium hydroxide | E558 - Bentonite (A natural type of clay from volcanic origin. It is a decolorising agent, filter medium, emulsifier and anti caking agent. Bentonite is used in pharmaceutical agents for external use, edible fats and oils, sugar, wine.) |
| E508 - Potassium chloride | E527 - Ammonium hydroxide | E559 – Kaolin |
| E509 - Calcium chloride | E528 - Magnesium hydroxide | E570 - Stearic acid |
| E510 - Ammonium chloride | E529 - Calcium oxide | E572 - Magnesium stearate, calcium stearate |
| E511 - Magnesium chloride | E530 - Magnesium oxide | E574 - Gluconic acid |
| E512 - Stannous chloride | E535 - Sodium ferrocyanide | E575 - Glucono delta-lactone |
| E513 - Sulphuric acid | E536 - Ptassium ferrocyanide | E576 - Sodium gluconate |
| E514 - Sodium sulphates | E538 - Calcium ferrocyanide | E577 - Potassium gluconate |
| E515 - Potassium sulphate | E540 - Dicalcium diphosphate | E578 - Calcium gluconate |
| E516 - Calcium sulphate | E541 - Sodium aluminium phosphate | E579 - Ferrous gluconate |
| E517 - Ammonium sulphate | E542 - Bone phosphate, edible bone phosphate (derived from steaming animal bones and used as anti caking agent, emulsifier and source of phosphorous in food supplements.) | E585 - Ferrous lactate |
| E518 - Magnesium sulphate, Epsom salts | E550 - Sodium silicate | E900 – Polydimethylsiloxane |
| E519 - Copper sulphate | E551 - Silicon dioxide | E553(a) - (i) Magnesium silicate and (ii) magnesium trisilicate |
| E520 - Aluminium sulphate | E552 - Calcium silicate | E553(b) – Talc |

# Food Coloring

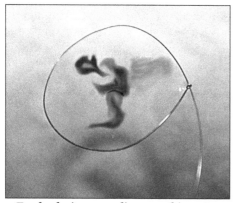

Food coloring spreading on a thin water film in the International Space Station.

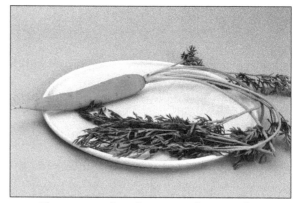

The orange color of carrots and many other fruits and vegetables arises from carotenoids.

Food coloring, or color additive, is any dye, pigment or substance that imparts color when it is added to food or drink. They come in many forms consisting of liquids, powders, gels, and pastes. Food coloring is used both in commercial food production and in domestic cooking. Food colorants are also used in a variety of non-food applications including cosmetics, pharmaceuticals, home craft projects, and medical devices.

## Purpose of Food Coloring

People associate certain colors with certain flavors, and the color of food can influence the perceived flavor in anything from candy to wine. Sometimes the aim is to simulate a color that is perceived by the consumer as natural, such as adding red coloring to glacé cherries (which would otherwise be beige), but sometimes it is for effect, like the green ketchup that Heinz launched in 1999. Color additives are used in foods for many reasons including:

- To make food more attractive, appealing, appetizing, and informative.

- Offset color loss due to exposure to light, air, temperature extremes, moisture and storage conditions.

- Correct natural variations in color.

- Enhance colors that occur naturally.

- Provide color to colorless and "fun" foods.

- Allow consumers to identify products on sight, like candy flavors or medicine dosages.

## Natural Food Dyes

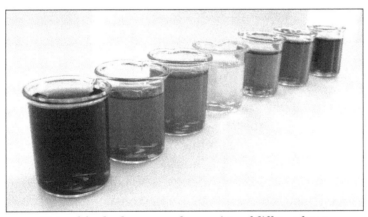

Natural food colors can make a variety of different hues.

Carotenoids (E160, E161, E164), chlorophyllin (E140, E141), anthocyanins (E163), and betanin (E162) comprise four main categories of plant pigments grown to color food products. Other colorants or specialized derivatives of these core groups include:

- Annatto (E160b), a reddish-orange dye made from the seed of the achiote,

- Caramel coloring (E150a-d), made from caramelized sugar,

- Carmine (E120), a red dye derived from the cochineal insect, Dactylopius coccus,

- Elderberry juice (E163),

- Lycopene (E160d),

- Paprika (E160c),

- Turmeric (E100).

Blue colors are especially rare. One feasible blue dye currently in use is derived from spirulina. Some recent research has explored associating anthocyanins with other phenolics or aluminium ions to develop blue colors. However, the inherent problems posed by the nature of the food matrix, and the need for long-term stability, makes this a very difficult objective. The pigment genipin, present in the fruit of Gardenia jasminoides, can be treated with amino acids to produce the blue pigment gardenia blue.

To ensure reproducibility, the colored components of these substances are often provided in highly purified form. For stability and convenience, they can be formulated in suitable carrier materials (solid and liquids). Hexane, acetone, and other solvents break down cell walls in the fruit and vegetables and allow for maximum extraction of the coloring. Traces of these may still remain in the finished colorant, but they do not need to be declared on the product label. These solvents are known as carry-over ingredients.

## Health Implications

Widespread public belief that artificial food coloring causes ADHD-like hyperactivity in children originated from Benjamin Feingold, a pediatric allergist from California, who proposed in 1973 that salicylates, artificial colors, and artificial flavors cause hyperactivity in children; however, there is no evidence to support broad claims that food coloring causes food intolerance and ADHD-like behavior in children. It is possible that certain food colorings may act as a trigger in those who are genetically predisposed, but the evidence is weak.

Despite concerns expressed that food colorings may cause ADHD-like behavior in children, the collective evidence does not support this assertion. The US FDA and other food safety authorities regularly review the scientific literature, and led the UK Food Standards Agency (FSA) to commission a study by researchers at Southampton University of the effect of a mixture of six food dyes (Tartrazine, Allura Red, Ponceau 4R, Quinoline Yellow WS, Sunset Yellow and Carmoisine (dubbed the "Southampton 6")) on children in the general population. These colorants are found in beverages. The study found "a possible link between the consumption of these artificial colors and a sodium benzoate preservative and increased hyperactivity" in the children; the advisory committee to the FSA that evaluated the study also determined that because of study limitations, the results could not be extrapolated to the general population, and further testing was recommended. The U.S. FDA did not make changes following the publication of the Southampton study. Following a citizen petition filed by the Center for Science in the Public Interest in 2008, requesting the FDA ban several food additives, the FDA reviewed the available evidence, and still made no changes.

The European regulatory community, with an emphasis on the precautionary principle, required labelling and temporarily reduced the acceptable daily intake (ADI) for the food colorings; the UK FSA called for voluntary withdrawal of the colorings by food manufacturers. However, in 2009 the EFSA re-evaluated the data at hand and determined that "the available scientific evidence does not substantiate a link between the color additives and behavioral effects" for any of the dyes.

## Chemical Structures of Representative Colorants

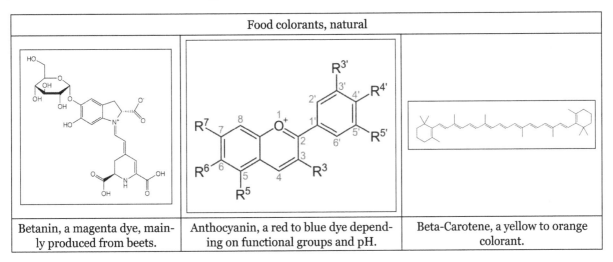

| Food colorants, natural | | |
| --- | --- | --- |
| Betanin, a magenta dye, mainly produced from beets. | Anthocyanin, a red to blue dye depending on functional groups and pH. | Beta-Carotene, a yellow to orange colorant. |

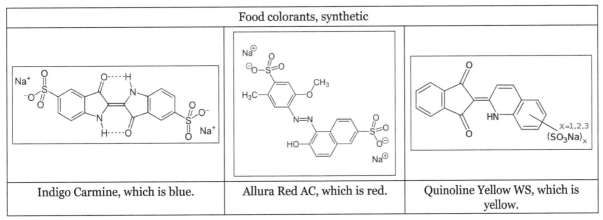

| Food colorants, synthetic | | |
| --- | --- | --- |
| Indigo Carmine, which is blue. | Allura Red AC, which is red. | Quinoline Yellow WS, which is yellow. |

# Humectants

A humectant is a hygroscopic substance used to keep things moist. It is often a molecule with several hydrophilic groups, most often hydroxyl groups; however, amines and carboxyl groups, sometimes esterified, can be encountered as well (its affinity to form hydrogen bonds with molecules of water is the crucial trait). They are used in many products, including food, cosmetics, medicines and pesticides.

A humectant attracts and retains the moisture in the air nearby via absorption, drawing the water vapor into or beneath the organism's or object's surface. This is the opposite use of a hygroscopic material where it is used as a desiccant used to draw moisture away.

When used as a food additive, a humectant has the effect of keeping moisture in the food.

Examples of some humectants include:

- Propylene glycol, hexylene glycol, and butylene glycol,

- Aloe vera gel,

- Alpha hydroxy acids such as lactic acid,

- Egg yolk and egg white,

- Glyceryl triacetate,

- Honey,

- Lithium chloride,

- Molasses,

- Polymeric polyols such as polydextrose,

- Quillaia,

- Sodium hexametaphosphate E452i,

- Sugar alcohols (sugar polyols) such as glycerol, sorbitol, xylitol, maltitol,

- Urea,

- Castor oil.

## Uses

A humectant is a substance that is used to keep products moisturized and affects the preservation of items, which can be used in, food and tobacco.

Some common humectants used in food are honey and glucose syrup both for their water absorption and sweet flavor. Glucose syrup also helps to retain the shape of the product better than other alternatives, for a longer period of time. In addition, some humectants are recognized in different countries as good food additives because of the increase in nutritional value that they provide, such as sodium hexametaphosphate.

In order to gauge a compound's humectancy, scientists will put it through a series of tests, often involving water absorption. In tests involving toothpaste, the process is also coupled with a sweetness test and a crystallization test. When humectancy is being assessed in different products, testers will compare the results to other humectants that are already used in those products, in order to evaluate efficiency.

Some of these humectants are seen in non-ionic polyols like sucrose, glycerin or glycerol and its triester (triacetin). These humectant food additives are used for the purpose of controlling viscosity and texture. Humectants also add bulk, retain moisture, reduce water activity, and improve softness. A main advantage of humectant food additives is that, since they are non-ionic, they are not expected to influence any variation of the pH aqueous systems.

Glycerol or glycerin humectants undergo a pretreatment process using saponification, bleaching, ion exchange exclusion, both cationic and ionic ion exchanges, vacuum flash evaporation, thin film distillation, and heating to produce a 100% pure glycerol.

Humectants are used in stabilization of food products and lengthening shelf life through food and moisture control. The available moisture determines microbial activity, physical properties, sensory properties and the rate of chemical changes, that if not controlled, are the cause of reduced shelf life. Examples are dry cereal with semi-moist raisins, ice cream in a cone, chocolate, hard candy with liquid centers and cheese. Humectants are used to stabilize the moisture content of foodstuffs and are incorporated as food additives. Humectants are also used in military technology for the use of MREs and other military rations. A number of food items always need to be moist. The use of humectants reduces the available water, thus reducing bacterial activity. They are used for safety issues, for quality, and to have a longer shelf-life in food products.

An example of where humectants are used to keep food moist is in products like toothpaste as well as certain kinds of cookies. Regional kinds of cookies often use humectants as a binding agent in order to keep moisture locked into the center of the cookie rather than have it evaporate out. Humectants are favored in food products because of their ability to keep consumable goods moist and increase shelf-life.

## Flavorings

Flavorings are intense preparations which are added to foods in order to impart taste and/or smell. These food flavors are used in small amounts and are not intended to be consumed alone. There are certain natural food flavors which are derived from herbs, spices and substances having an exclusively sweet, sour or salt taste.

### Types of Food Flavoring

Flavorings are used as food additives for altering and/or enhancing the flavors of natural food products. Sometimes, food flavorings are also used to create flavor for food products that do not have desired flavors such as candies and other snacks. There are three major types of food flavorings that are used in foods. These types of flavorings are mostly used as criteria for food regulatory purposes in European Union and Australia. In North America, the classification of flavorings is done as - Natural flavorings and Synthetic flavorings. The Synthetic flavorings there include both artificial and nature-identical flavorings.

- Natural flavoring substances: Flavoring substances that are obtained from plant or animal raw materials, by physical, microbiological or enzymatic processes are classified as natural flavoring substances. These natural flavorings can be either used in their natural form or processed form for consumption by human beings. However, they cannot contain any nature-identical or artificial flavoring substances.

- Nature-identical flavoring substances: Nature-identical substances are the flavoring substances that are obtained by synthesis or are isolated through chemical processes, which are chemically identical to flavoring substances naturally present in products intended for consumption by human beings. These flavorings cannot contain any artificial flavoring substances.

- Artificial flavoring substances: Flavoring substances that are not identified in a natural product intended for consumption by human being- whether or not the product is processed- are artificial flavoring substances. These food flavorings are typically produced by fractional distillation and additional chemical manipulation naturally sourced chemicals or from crude oil or coal tar.

## Chemicals Associated with Particular Flavors

| Allylpyrazine | Flavor |
|---|---|
| Color | Roasted nut |
| Methoxypyrazines | Earthy vegetables |
| 2-Isobutyl-3 Methoxypyrazine | Green pepper |
| Acetyl-L-Pyrazines | Popcorn |
| Aldehydes | Fruity, green |
| Alcohols | Bitter, medicinal |
| Esters | Fruity |
| Ketones | Butter, caramel |
| Pyrazines | Brown, burnt, caramel, |
| Phenolics | Medicinal, smokey |
| Terpenoids | Citrus, piney |

## Smoke Flavoring Substances

Although it is not one of the basic flavorings, smoke flavoring has come up as a significant food flavoring substance in the world of food additives. Smoke flavoring is a natural flavoring concentrate obtained by subjecting untreated and uncontaminated hardwood, including sawdust and woody plants, to one or more of these listed processes for obtaining fractions which have the desired flavor potential.

- Controlled burning,

- Dry distillation at appropriate temperatures,

- Treatment with superheated steam.

As per the above classification, we get three types of flavorings- natural flavorings, nature identical flavoring and artificial flavoring. There is also a difference for regulation of natural food flavoring in the US and EU that can be made clear by the definitions provided by the food laws of both the regions.

## Basic Food Flavors

There are three basic parameters based on which all food flavorings are made. These three components of food flavors are- smell, taste and color.

## Flavoring Smell

Making of flavoring smells or odors are similar to the making process of industrial fragrances and perfumes. To make natural flavors with desired smell, the flavorant is extracted from the source substance through various methods like solvent extraction, distillation, or using force to squeeze it out. These extracts are then further purified and added to food products in order to give them a particular flavor. To make artificial flavors, the individual naturally occurring aroma chemicals are identified and then mixed to produce a desired flavor. These mixtures are formulated by flavor chemist or flavorist to give a food product a unique flavor and to maintain flavor consistency between different product batches or after recipe changes.

## Flavoring Tastes

There are four basic tastes known to human beings- sweet, sour, salty, and bitter. The substances that enhance umami and other secondary flavors are considered to be taste flavorants. The dictionary defines umami as- "a taste that is characteristic of monosodium glutamate and is associated with meats and other high-protein foods. It is sometimes considered to be a fifth basic taste along with sweet, sour, salty, and bitter." Therefore flavoring tastes can be identified with flavor enhancers that are largely based on amino acids and nucleotides and are typically used as sodium or calcium salts. Some of the Umami flavorants recognized and approved by the European Union include:

- Glutamic acid salts,
- Glycine salts,
- Guanylic acid salts,
- Nucleotide salts,
- Inosinic acid salts,
- 5'-ribonucleotide salts.

## Flavoring Colors

The color of food also affects its flavor. Therefore, food flavor suppliers have all kinds of flavoring colors with them. Food colorings are derived from natural sources as well as from chemicals. The flavoring color additive regulations around the world are different from each other. Certain food colors that are permitted to be used in Europe or Asia may not be acceptable in the United States and vice versa.

## Thickeners and Vegetable Gums

### Food Thickeners

Thickening agents, or thickeners, are substances that are added to food preparations for increasing their viscosity without changing other properties like taste.

The food thickeners are the modified food starch, polysaccharide or certain vegetable gums. When a food thickener or a thickening agent is added to beverage, it absorbs the fluid and the fluid thickens. Breaking down the starch reverses the thickening action and almost all water in the beverage is available as free fluid for absorption by the body. If the thickening agent is a vegetable gum, it will continue to hold water even during digestion. Thus a vegetable based thickening agent may reduce fluid availability to the body. Commonly used thickening agents are pectin, lignin, algin, gums and agar-agar.

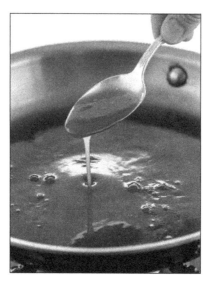

## Use of Food Thickening Agent

The use of food thickening agents depends upon the type of food and purpose for which you are going to use them. For example, for acidic foods, use of arrowroot as a thickening agent is preferred instead of cornstarch as the later loses the thickening property in acidic food. Some of the food thickeners can be used any time during the cooking of food and some are used close to the final stage.

Flour is a food thickening agent that is used in between the cooking as it needs to be prepared otherwise it will give uncooked taste. For gravies, sauces and stews, Raux is used as a food thickener. Raux is typically made from flour and butter. This food thickener is used while making thick gravy. Egg yolks, nuts, yogurts are some other natural food thickeners that are used as food thickening agents.

## Types of Food Thickener

Food thickener when used in any food absorbs the fluid to thicken it but does not change the physical or chemical properties of the food. Based on how and from which these are made the food thickeners are classified into two categories. These are:

- Polysaccharides (starches, vegetable gums, and pectin),
- Proteins.

Polysaccharides as a thickener food includes the starches, vegetable gums and pectin. Food starch is a flavorless powder in which can be included arrowroot, cornstarch, katakuri starch, potato starch, sago, and tapioca.

## Using Food Thickeners

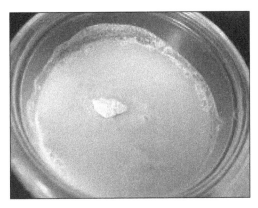

How to use a food thickener is generally mentioned on the packing. You can thicken the sauces and vegetables by putting the food thickener in them. Now the amount of the food thickeners required actually depends upon the value of thickness needed. Also the property of food thickening agent should be considered to thicken the food. Along with this the way to use the food thickening agent will make the changes. Like all of us use custard powder to make custard that also has the food thickening agent. If you will stir it while cooking then it will be like a sauce. But not stirring it will result into thick custard that can be sliced like jelly.

You need constant stirring if using flour as a food thickener. If not stirred, lumps will be created that are then very difficult to dissolve. Also before using it first make its mixture in water or liquid you are going to use and then cook it in gravy or food.

Eggs are also used as food thickener for sauces. It is a protein based food thickener so will coagulate giving your sauce or soup a coagulated look.

You can use the thickeners and vegetable gums with all kinds of food colors like natural food color, synthetic food color and lake food colors.

## Food Thickening Gums

One of the types of food thickeners are gums. All gums are polysaccharides, that is similar to sugars but with many sugar units making up a large molecule. They are bland in taste, odour less and tasteless. They may have a nutritional quality besides the primary function but they certainly help in digestion and may be used as laxatives too. Vegetable gums used as food thickeners include alginin, guar gum, locust bean gum, and xanthan gum.

## Vegetable Gums

Vegetable gums come from the varied sources that can be on land or in sea. Some of the seaweeds are the excellent sources of food gums in which comes the carrageenan and alginates. Whereas guar, locust bean gum, pectin are obtained from the plants. Xanthan gum is obtained by the process of microbial fermentation. The source of gelatin is animal tissue.

Vegetable gums are the polysaccharides that have the natural origin and used to increase the viscosity of the solution or food even if used in a very small concentration.

So vegetable gums are actually the food thickening agents.

- Major vegetable gums,

- Xanthan vegetable gum,

- Xanthan gum,

- Agar agar,

- Cellulose gum,

- Xanthan gum,

- Guar gum,

- Locust bean gum,

- Pectin.

Agar Agar agar is used as a vegetable gum for gelling the dairy products like yogurt. Agar agar as a food thickener has the capacity to absorb 100 times more water than its weight. Agar agar is a polysaccharide that has the repeating unit of alpha-D-galactopyranosyl and 3,6-anhydro-alpha-L-glactopyranosyl.

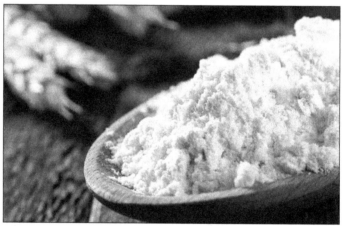

Xanthan gum.

Cellulose Gum Use of cellulose gum as a vegetable gum and food thickening agent is not new. At home homemakers have been using it for the last 50 years. All cellulose vegetable gums are water soluble because of the cellulose content in it. It is used in ice-creams, beverages and in baked food products to prevent stalling. Also the ice-crystal formulation in ice-creams is prevented by this vegetable gum.

Xanthan Gum Xanthan Gum is again a polysaccharide and chiefly used in salad dressing and sauces. Also some of the bakery filling use the Xanthan gum that is an excellent food thickener. This vegetable gum is also used to increase the shelf period of eatables.

Guar Gum is a carbohydrate based vegetable gum and food thickener that swell up in cold water. It is an excellent food thickening agent used in food industry as it has about 80-85% of soluble dietary fibers. Because of this reason guar gum is also used in bread to have more soluble dietary content.

Locust Bean Gum Locust Bean Gum is also called the Carob bean gum as it is made from the carob bean's seed. It is mainly used in food for water binding, thickening and gel strengthening. This vegetable gum is used as dessert gel, dairy applications and as processed cream cheese.

Pectin is a kind of polysaccharide that is obtained from plant such as citrus fruit peel, apple peel etc. Pectin is a vegetable gum and food thickener that is used to make gel. You will find in almost every fruit based product such as jam, confectioneries, fruit drinks etc. Apart from this yogurt and other dairy products also use this vegetable gum as food thickener.

# Leavening Agents

A leaven, often called a leavening agent (and also known as a raising agent) is any one of a number of substances used in doughs and batters that cause a foaming action (gas bubbles) that lightens and softens the mixture. An alternative or supplement to leavening agents is mechanical action by which air is incorporated. Leavening agents can be biological or synthetic chemical compounds. The gas produced is often carbon dioxide, or occasionally hydrogen.

When a dough or batter is mixed, the starch in the flour and the water in the dough form a matrix (often supported further by proteins like gluten or polysaccharides, such as pentosans or xanthan gum). Then the starch gelatinizes and sets, leaving gas bubbles that remain.

## Biological Leavening Agents

- Saccharomyces cerevisiae producing carbon dioxide found in:
  - Baker's yeast,
  - beer (unpasteurised—live yeast),
  - ginger beer,
  - kefir,
  - sourdough starter.
- *Clostridium perfringens* producing hydrogen found in salt-rising bread.

## Chemical Leavens

Chemical leavens are mixtures or compounds that release gases when they react with each other, with moisture, or with heat. Most are based on a combination of acid (usually a low molecular weight organic acid) and a salt of bicarbonate ($HCO_3^-$). After they act, these compounds leave behind a chemical salt. Chemical leavens are used in quick breads and cakes, as well as cookies and numerous other applications where a long biological fermentation is impractical or undesirable.

## Other Leavens

Steam and air are used as leavening agents when they expand upon heating. To take advantage of this style of leavening, the baking must be done at high enough temperatures to flash the water to steam, with a batter that is capable of holding the steam in until set. This effect is typically used in popovers, Yorkshire puddings, and to a lesser extent in tempura.

Nitrous oxide is used as a propellant in aerosol whip cream cans. Large densities of $N_2O$ are dissolved in cream at high pressure. When expelled from the can, the nitrous oxide escapes emulsion instantly, creating a temporary foam in the butterfat matrix of the cream.

## Mechanical Leavening

Creaming is the process of beating sugar crystals and solid fat (typically butter) together in a mixer. This integrates tiny air bubbles into the mixture, since the sugar crystals physically cut through the structure of the fat. Creamed mixtures are usually further leavened by a chemical leaven like baking soda. This is often used in cookies.

Using a whisk on certain liquids, notably cream or egg whites, can also create foams through mechanical action. This is the method employed in the making of sponge cakes, where an egg protein matrix produced by vigorous whipping provides almost all the structure of the finished product.

The Chorleywood bread process uses a mix of biological and mechanical leavening to produce bread; while it is considered by food processors to be an effective way to deal with the soft wheat flours characteristic of British Isles agriculture, it is controversial due to a perceived lack of quality in the final product. The process has nevertheless been adapted by industrial bakers in other parts of the world.

## Glazing Agents

Glazing Agents are "substances which, when applied to the external surface of a foodstuff, impart a shiny appearance or provide a protective coating".

## Source

Many glazing agents and edible surface coatings are derived from waxes naturally produced by animals and plants to retain moisture, while others are synthetically derived from petroleum. Some of the main food glazing agents are.

| E Number | Product |
|---|---|
| E901 | Beeswax, white and yellow, produced by honey bees. |
| E902 | Candelilla wax, from the Mexican shrubs Euphorbia cerifera and Euphorbia antisyphilitica. |
| E903 | Carnauba wax, from the leaves of the Carnauba palm, Copernicia cerifera or the Brazilian palm, Copernicia prunifera. |
| E904 | Shellac, a wax-containing resin secreted by the Lac insect Kerria lacca. |
| E905 | Microcrystalline wax, produced by de-oiling Petrolatum. |

## Properties

Surface coatings are applied as a powder or liquid layer onto a product via mechanical processes such as spraying, mixing or dipping. Having uniformly applied the coating to the product, the coating is stabilised by drying, heating, cooling or freezing, helping to prolong the product's longevity. Encapsulation involves the application of a liquid layer to minute particles and relies on more processes than mechanical movement alone, such as entrapping a molecule inside a matrix, polymerisation and chemical bonding.

Glazing agents create a glossy, smooth surface coating that provides a protective, moisture resistant barrier. The coating helps to preserve food products by locking-in internal moisture or preventing their degradation due to external humidity, resulting in a prolonged shelf-life. Desirable properties of glazing agents include the stability to maintain their integrity under heat or pressure and their ability to provide a uniform, homogenous coating on an industrial scale.

## Uses

### Food Industry

Surface coatings are used to enhance the aesthetic appeal of food products by improving their lustre or changing their color. They can also improve the palatability of the products by changing their texture or taste, or by enhancing their flavor. Surface coatings are sometimes used to enrich the product by adding vitamins and minerals. They may also function as release agents to prevent packaging sticking to the products.

### Confectionery Industry

Confectionery products are often coated by sugar panning, which involves tumbling products such as nuts, chocolates or jelly beans in a syrup to create a sugary outer shell. Confectioner's glaze is often used to provide a glossy surface coating for candies.

## References

- Food-additive, topic: britannica.com, Retrieved 16 July, 2019
- Anticaking-agents: foodadditivesworld.com, Retrieved 02 June, 2019
- Flavorings: foodadditivesworld.com, Retrieved 25 March, 2019
- Thickeners-and-vegetable-gums: foodadditivesworld.com, Retrieved 05 May, 2019
- Glazing-agents-edible-surface-coatings, application: afsuter.com, Retrieved 18 January, 2019
- Ian P. Freeman, "Margarines and Shortenings" Ullmann's Encyclopedia of Industrial Chemistry, 2005, Wiley-VCH, Weinheim doi:10.1002/14356007.a16_145

# 5

# Food Contamination

Food contamination is the presence of harmful chemicals and microorganisms in food which can cause food-borne illnesses. Biological contamination, physical contamination, chemical contamination, etc. fall under its domain. The topics elaborated in this chapter will help in gaining a better perspective about these aspects related to food contamination.

Food contamination is generally defined as foods that are spoiled or tainted because they either contain microorganisms, such as bacteria or parasites, or toxic substances that make them unfit for consumption. A food contaminant can be biological, chemical or physical in nature, with the former being more common. These contaminants have several routes throughout the supply chain (farm to fork) to enter and make a food product unfit for consumption. Bacillus cereus, Campylobacter jejuni, Clostridium botulinum, C. perfrigens, Pathogenic Escherichia coli, Listeria monocytogenes, Salmonella spp., Shigellaspp., Pathogenic Staphylococcus aureus, Vibrio cholera, V. parahaemolyticus, V. vulnificus and Yersinia enterocolitica are common bacterial hazards (a type of biological contaminant). Chemical food contaminants that can enter the food supply chain include pesticides, heavy metals, and other alien chemical agents.

The World Health Organization (WHO) has recognized food contamination as a global challenge in several documents and reports. It is clearly acknowledged in a statement: "Food contamination that occurs in one place may affect the health of consumers living on the other side of the planet". In fact, a vast majority of people experience a foodborne or waterborne disease at some point in their lives worldwide. Therefore, consumption of contaminated foods causes illness in millions of people and many die as a result of it. This scenario makes "food contamination" a serious issue. The list of food contamination challenges is very long and keeps growing.

Contamination of fresh produce is emerging as a major food safety challenge. A recent report by the Center for Science in the Public Interest (CSPI) showed that the highest number of outbreaks was attributed to produce as a single commodity in the USA during 2002–2011. Similarly, produce caused the greatest number of illnesses and the largest average number of illnesses per outbreak. This is a global trend and can be seen in examples of recent outbreaks: an outbreak of E. coli O157:H7 after eating contaminated packaged baby spinach in the EU; E. coli in cucumber outbreak in Germany and other EU countries; an outbreak of Cryptosporidium infection traced to bagged salads in the UK; an outbreak of L. monocytogenes due to contaminated prepacked salad products, and a Salmonella outbreak linked to lettuce in pre-packaged salads in Australia.

The emergence of antibiotic resistance bacteria (ARB) is now accepted a potential threat to both public and environmental health and the WHO has already proposed a global strategy to address the challenge. Publications describing the association and prevalence of ARB in food products are common now. Previously the clinical arena was the major culprit; however, the overuse of antibiotics in food production is making the situation more complicated. In brief, foods contaminated with ARB are going to be a major food safety issue in the future.

Intentional contamination of foods and food products is also a growing global concern. Intentional food contamination refers to the deliberate addition of a harmful or poisonous substance to food products. It is a criminal act and also known as food fraud. Foods that have been intentionally contaminated are unsafe to eat and can make consumers seriously ill. Therefore, it is also equally important to address the challenge of fraudulent food contamination.

Food safety is generally compromised when food products get contaminated with a potentially hazardous and toxic agent. The food industry faces many global, as well as regional, contamination issues, existing and emerging, at all times, and continues to address them through scientific and technological developments. Therefore, it is vital for food safety management to understand the nature of contamination, its sources, risks to the consumer, and approaches to eliminate or reduce contamination levels. Sound scientific knowledge is needed to provide food products that are free of contamination or with a minimal risk of contamination.

# Food Contaminants

Food contamination refers to the presence of harmful chemicals and microorganisms in food, which can cause consumer illness.

The impact of chemical contaminants on consumer health and well-being is often apparent only after many years of processing and prolonged exposure at low levels (e.g., cancer). Unlike food-borne pathogens, chemical contaminants present in foods are often unaffected by thermal processing. Chemical contaminants can be classified according to the source of contamination and the mechanism by which they enter the food product.

## Agrochemicals

Agrochemicals are chemicals used in agricultural practices and animal husbandry with the intent to increase crop yields. Such agents include pesticides (e.g., insecticides, herbicides, rodenticides), plant growth regulators, veterinary drugs (e.g., nitrofuran, fluoroquinolones, malachite green, chloramphenicol), and bovine somatotropin (rBST).

## Environmental Contaminants

Environmental contaminants are chemicals that are present in the environment in which the food is grown, harvested, transported, stored, packaged, processed, and consumed. The physical contact of the food with its environment results in its contamination. Possible sources of contamination and contaminants common to that vector include:

- Air: Radionuclides (caesium-137, strontium-90), polycyclic aromatic hydrocarbons (PAH).

- Water: Arsenic, mercury.

- Soil: Cadmium, nitrates, perchlorates.

- Packaging materials: Antimony, tin, lead, perfluorooctanoic acid (PFOA), semicarbazide, benzophenone, isopropylthioxanthone (ITX), bisphenol A.

- Processing/cooking equipment: Copper or other metal chips, lubricants, cleaning and sanitizing agents.

- Naturally occurring toxins: Mycotoxins, phytohemagglutinin, pyrrolizidine alkaloids, grayanotoxin, mushroom toxins, scombrotoxin (histamine), ciguatera, shellfish toxins, tetrodotoxin, among many others.

## Pesticides and Carcinogens

There are many cases of banned pesticides or carcinogens found in foods:

- Greenpeace exposed in 2006 that 25% of surveyed supermarkets in China stocked agricultural products contaminated with banned pesticides. Over 70% of tomatoes that tested were found to have the banned pesticide Lindane, and almost 40% of the samples had a mix of three or more types of pesticides. Tangerine, strawberry, and Kyofung grape samples were also found contaminated by banned pesticides, including the highly toxic methamidophos. Greenpeace says there exists no comprehensive monitoring on fruit produce in the Hong Kong as of 2006.

- In India, soft drinks were found contaminated with high levels of pesticides and insecticides, including lindane, DDT, malathion and chlorpyrifos.

- Formaldehyde, a carcinogen, was frequently found in the common Vietnamese dish, Pho, resulting in the 2007 Vietnam food scare. "Health agencies have known that Vietnamese soy sauce, the country's second most popular sauce after fish sauce, has been chock full of cancer agents since at least 2001", reported the *Thanh Nien* daily. "Why didn't anyone tell us?" The carcinogen in Asian sauces is 3-MCPD and its metabolite 1,3-DCP, which has been an ongoing problem affecting multiple continents. Vietnamese vegetables and fruits were also found to have banned pesticides.

- The 2005 Indonesia food scare, where carcinogenic formaldehyde was found to be added as a preservative to noodles, tofu, salted fish, and meatballs.

- In 2008 Chinese milk scandal, melamine was discovered to have been added to milk and infant formula which caused 54,000 babies to be sent to the hospital. Six babies died because of kidney stones related to the contaminant.

## Hair in Food

There is a heavy stigma attached to the presence of hair in food in most societies. There is a risk that it may induce choking and vomiting, and also that it may be contaminated by toxic substances. Views differ as to the level of risk it poses to the inadvertent consumer.

In most countries, people working in the food industry are required to cover their hair because it will contaminate the food. When people are served food which contains hair in restaurants or cafés, it is usual for them to complain to the staff.

There are a range of possible reasons for the objection to hair in food, ranging from cultural taboos to the simple fact that it is difficult to digest and unpleasant to eat. It may also be interpreted as a sign of more widespread problems with hygiene. The introduction of complete-capture hairnets is believed to have resulted in a decrease in incidents of contamination of this type.

Sometimes protein from human hair is used as a food ingredient, in bread and other such similar products. Such use of human hair in food is forbidden in Islam. Historically, in Judaism, finding hair in food was a sign of bad luck.

## Processing Contaminants

Processing contaminants are generated during the processing of foods (e.g., heating, fermentation). They are absent in the raw materials, and are formed by chemical reactions between natural and/or added food constituents during processing. The presence of these contaminants in processed foods cannot be entirely avoided. Technological processes can be adjusted and/or optimized, however, in order to reduce the levels of formation of processing contaminants. Examples are: nitrosamines, polycyclic aromatic hydrocarbons (PAH), heterocyclic amines, histamine, acrylamide, furan, benzene, trans fat, 3-MCPD, semicarbazide, 4-hydroxynonenal (4-HNE), and ethyl carbamate. There is also the possibility of metal chips from the processing equipment contaminating food. These can be identified using metal detection equipment. In many conveyor lines, the line will be stopped, or when weighing the product with a Check weigher, the item can be rejected for being over- or underweight or because small pieces of metal are detected within it.

## Emerging Food Contaminants

While many food contaminants have been known for decades, the formation and presence of certain chemicals in foods has been discovered relatively recently. These are the so-called emerging food contaminants like acrylamide, furan, benzene, perchlorate, perfluorooctanoic acid (PFOA), 3-monochloropropane-1,3-diol (3-MCPD), 4-hydroxynonenal, and (4-HNE).

## Safety and Regulation

Acceptable daily intake (ADI) levels and tolerable concentrations of contaminants in individual foods are determined on the basis of the "No Observed Adverse Effect Level" (NOAEL) in animal experiments, by using a safety factor (usually 100). The maximum concentrations of contaminants allowed by legislation are often well below toxicological tolerance levels, because such levels can often be reasonably achieved by using good agricultural and manufacturing practices.

Regulatory officials, in order to combat the dangers associated with foodborne viruses, are pursuing various possible measures:

- The EFSA published a report in 2011 on "scientific opinion regarding an update of the present knowledge on the occurrence and control of foodborne viruses".

- This year, an expert working group created by the European Committee for Standardization (CEN), is expected to publish a standard method for the detection of norovirus and hepatitis A virus in food.

- The CODEX Committee on Food Hygiene (CCFH) is also working on a guideline which is now ready for final adoption.

- European Commission Regulation (EC) No 2073/2005 of 15 November 2005 indicates that "foodstuffs should not contain micro-organisms or their toxins or metabolites in quantities that present an unacceptable risk for human health", underlining that methods are required for foodborne virus detection.

## Food Contaminant Testing

To maintain the high quality of food and comply with health, safety, and environmental regulatory standards, it is best to rely on food contaminant testing through an independent third party, such as laboratories or certification companies. For manufacturers, the testing for food contaminants can minimize the risk of noncompliance in relation to raw ingredients, semi-manufactured foods, and final products. Also, food contaminant testing assures consumers safety and quality of purchased food products and can prevent foodborne diseases, and chemical, microbiological, or physical food hazards.

The establishment of ADIs for certain emerging food contaminants is currently an active area of research and regulatory debate.

# Food Spoilage

Food spoilage is the process where a food product becomes unsuitable to ingest by the consumer. The cause of such a process is due to many outside factors as a side-effect of the type of product it is, as well as how the product is packaged and stored. Due to food spoilage, one-third of the worlds' food produced for the consumption of humans is lost every year. Bacteria and various fungi are the cause of spoilage and can create serious consequences for the consumers, but there are preventive measures that can be taken.

## Bacteria

Bacteria are responsible for the spoilage of food. When bacteria breaks down the food, acids and other waste products are created in the process. While the bacteria itself may or may not be harmful, the waste products may be unpleasant to taste or may even be harmful to one's health. There are two types of pathogenic bacteria that target different categories of food. The first type is called *Clostridium perfingens* and targets foods such as meat and poultry, and *Bacillus cereus*, which targets milk and cream. When stored or subjected to unruly conditions, the organisms will begin to breed apace, releasing harmful toxins that can cause severe illness, even when cooked safely.

## Fungi

*Fungi* has been seen as a method of food spoilage, causing only an undesirable appearance to food, however, there has been significant evidence of various fungi being a cause of death of many people spanning across hundreds of years in many places through the world. Fungi are caused by acidifying, fermenting, discoloring and disintegrating processes and can create fuzz, powder and slimes of many different colors, including black, white, red, brown and green.

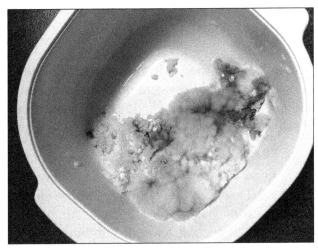

This image shows a bowl of white rice with mold growing over it.

*Mold* is a type of fungus, but the two terms are not reciprocal of each other; they have their own defining features and perform their own tasks. Very well-known types of mold are Aspergillus and Penicillium, and, like regular fungi, create a fuzz, powder and slime of various colors.

*Yeast* is also a type of fungus that grows vegetatively via single cells that either bud or divide by way of fission, allowing for yeast to multiply in liquid environments favoring the dissemination of single celled microorganisms. Yeast forms mainly in liquid environments and anaerobic conditions, but being single celled, it oftentimes cannot spread on or into solid surfaces where other fungus flourish. Yeast also produces at a slower rate than bacteria, therefore being at a disadvantage in environments where bacteria are. Yeasts can be responsible for the decomposition of food with a high sugar content. The same effect is useful in the production of various types of food and beverages, such as bread, yogurt, cider, and alcoholic beverages.

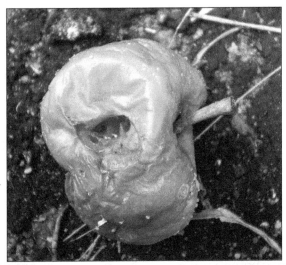

This image depicts the process of decomposition beyond the point of human appeal.

## Signs

Signs of food spoilage may include an appearance different from the food in its fresh form, such as a change in color, a change in texture, an unpleasant odour, or an undesirable taste. The item may become softer than normal. If mold occurs, it is often visible externally on the item.

## Consequences

Spoilage bacteria do not normally cause "food poisoning"; typically, the microorganisms that cause foodborne illnesses are odorless and flavorless, and otherwise undetectable outside the lab. Eating deteriorated food could not be considered safe due to mycotoxins or microbial wastes. Some pathogenic bacteria, such as *Clostridium perfringens* and *Bacillus cereus*, are capable of causing spoilage.

Issues of food spoilage do not necessarily have to do with the quality of the food, but more so with the safety of consuming said food. However, there are cases where food has been proven to contain toxic ingredients. 200 years ago, Claviceps purpurea, a type of fungus, was linked to human diseases and 100 years ago in Japan, yellow rice was found to contain toxic ingredients.

## Prevention

A number of methods of prevention can be used that can either totally prevent, delay, or otherwise reduce food spoilage. A food rotation system uses the first in first out method (FIFO), which ensures that the first item purchased is the first item consumed.

Preservatives can expand the shelf life of food and can lengthen the time long enough for it to be harvested, processed, sold, and kept in the consumer's home for a reasonable length of time. One of the age old techniques for food preservation, to avoid mold and fungus growth, is the process of drying out the food or dehydrating it. While there is a chance of it developing a fungus targeted towards dried food products, the chances are quite low.

Other than drying, other methods include salting, curing, canning, refrigeration, freezing, preservatives, irradiation, and high hydrostatic pressure: Refrigeration can increase the shelf life of certain foods and beverages, though with most items, it does not indefinitely expand it. Freezing can preserve food even longer, though even freezing has limitations. Canning of food can preserve food for a particularly long period of time, whether done at home or commercially. Canned food is vacuum packed in order to keep oxygen, which is needed by bacteria in aerobic spoilage, out of the can. Canning does have limitations, and does not preserve the food indefinitely. Lactic acid fermentation also preserves food and prevents spoilage.

Food like meat, poultry, milk and cream should be kept out of the Danger Zone (between 40°F to 140°F). Anything between that range is considered dangerous and can cause pathogenic toxins to be emitted, resulting in severe illness in the consumer. Another way to keep your food from spoiling is by following a four step system: Clean, Separate, Cook, Chill. This will reduce any risks.

## Benzene in Soft Drinks

Benzene in soft drinks is of potential concern due to the carcinogenic nature of the benzene molecule. This contamination is a public health concern and has caused significant outcry among environmental and health advocates. Benzene levels are regulated in drinking water nationally and internationally, and in bottled water in the United States, but only informally in soft drinks. The benzene forms from decarboxylation of the preservative benzoic acid in the presence of ascorbic acid (vitamin C) and metal ions (iron and copper) that act as catalysts, especially under heat and light.

## Formation in Soft Drinks

The major cause of benzene in soft drinks is the decarboxylation of benzoic acid in the presence of ascorbic acid (vitamin C, E300) or erythorbic acid (a diastereomer of ascorbic acid, E315). Benzoic acid is often added to drinks as a preservative in the form of its salts sodium benzoate (E211), potassium benzoate (E 212), or calcium benzoate (E 213). Citric acid is not thought to induce significant benzene production in combination with benzoic acid, but some evidence suggests that in the presence of ascorbic or erythorbic acid and benzoic acid, citric acid may accelerate the production of benzene.

The proposed mechanism begins with hydrogen abstraction by the hydroxyl radical, which itself is produced by the $Cu^{2+}$-catalysed reduction of dioxygen by ascorbic acid:

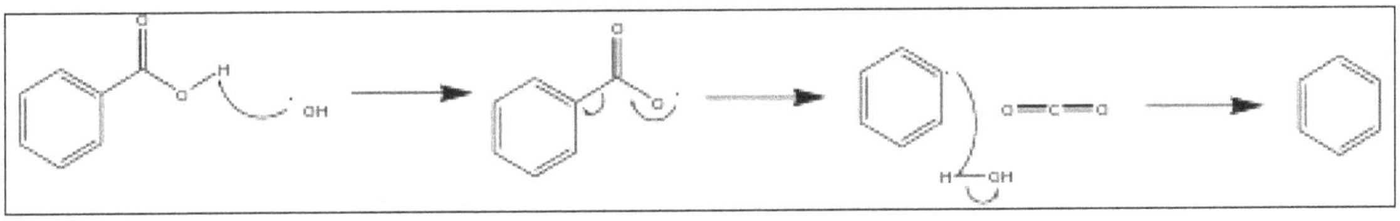

Other factors that affect the formation of benzene are heat and light. Storing soft drinks in warm conditions speeds up the formation of benzene.

Calcium disodium EDTA and sugars have been shown to inhibit benzene production in soft drinks.

The International Council of Beverages Associations (ICBA) has produced advice to prevent or minimize benzene formation.

## Limit Standards in Drinking Water

Various authorities have set limits on benzene content in drinking water. The following limits are given in parts per billion (ppb; µg/kg):

- World Health Organization (WHO): 10 ppb (WHO notes that benzene should be avoided whenever technically feasible),

- Republic of Korea (South Korea): 10 ppb,

- Canada: 5 ppb,

- United States: 5 ppb,

- European Union: 1 ppb,

- State limits within the United States: California, Connecticut, New Jersey, and Florida: 1 ppb.

The EPA and California have set public health goals for benzene of 0 ppb and 0.15 ppb.

## Environmental Exposure to Benzene

Benzene in soft drinks has to be seen in the context of other environmental exposure. Taking the worst example found to date of a soft drink containing 87.9 ppb benzene, someone drinking a 350 ml (12 oz) can would ingest 31 μg (micrograms) of benzene, almost equivalent to the benzene inhaled by a motorist refilling a fuel tank for three minutes. While there are alternatives to using sodium benzoate as a preservative, the casual consumption of such a drink is unlikely to pose a significant health hazard to a particular individual.

The UK Food Standards Agency has stated that people would need to drink at least 20 litres (5.5 gal) per day of a drink containing benzene at 10 μg to equal the amount of benzene they would breathe from city air every day. Daily personal exposure to benzene is determined by adding exposure from all sources.

- Air: A European study found that people breathe in 220 μg of benzene every day due to general atmospheric pollution. A motorist refilling a fuel tank for three minutes would inhale a further 32 μg. The estimated daily exposure from "automobile-related activities" is 49 μg and for driving for one hour is 40 μg.

- Smoking: For smokers, cigarette smoking is the main source of exposure to benzene. Estimates are 7900 μg per day (smoking 20 cigarettes per day), 1820 μg/day, and 1800 μg/day.

- Passive smoking: Benzene intake from passive smoking is estimated at 63 μg/day (Canada) and 50 μg/day.

- Diet and drinking water: 0.2 to 3.1 μg per day.

## Biological Contamination

Biological contamination is when bacteria or other harmful microorganisms contaminate food; it is a common cause of food poisoning and food spoilage.

Food poisoning can happen when disease-causing bacteria or other germs, also called 'pathogens', spread to food and are consumed. Bacteria are small microorganisms that split and multiply very quickly. In conditions ideal for bacterial growth, one single-cell bacteria can become two million in just seven hours.

Certain types of bacteria also produce bacterial toxins in the process of multiplying and producing waste. Bacterial toxins can be very dangerous — in fact, botulinum, the bacterial toxin that causes botulism, is the most potent natural poison known.

Certain foods are more vulnerable to biological contamination than others because they provide everything bacteria need to survive and multiply — food, water and neutral acidity (pH). These are called high-risk foods. When high-risk foods are left in the Temperature Danger Zone (5 °C – 60 °C) for too long, Food Handlers provide the other conditions bacteria need to grow — time and the right temperature.

It's important to remember that all foods can harbour dangerous pathogens. Norovirus, for example, doesn't grow or multiply on food, but it can survive for days or even weeks on any type of food and is a leading cause of food-borne illness.

# Physical Contamination

Physical contamination happens when actual objects contaminate foods. Sometimes when a food is physically contaminated, it can also be biologically contaminated. This is because the physical contamination might harbour dangerous bacteria, for example, a fingernail.

Ingestion of a piece of a hard or sharp material such as glass or metal could cause an unsuspecting consumer severe injury, require surgery, or have deadly consequences. Therefore, food contamination has always been a major concern of the food industry, and consumers.

Most physical contaminants of foods, such as pieces of hard plastic or wood, can cause consumers immediate injury; this includes all types of foods, including beverages, bottled water, and nutritional and functional products. Any physical material in food that does not belong in the product may be classified as a physical contaminant.

Physical contaminants are also referred to as physical hazards or foreign matter. Shrew teeth in a crop product or a piece of wire in a meat product are examples. Glass pieces, metal fragments, bone chips, and pits may all cause serious harm when ingested. Common examples of bodily harm include lacerations of the lips, the inside of the mouth, teeth, gums, tongue, throat, esophagus, stomach, and intestine, and even choking. Children and seniors are at greater risk and have the highest incidence of such harm.

Government agencies, food producers, manufacturers, distributors, and retailers must all protect the health of the consumer as one of their most important objectives and responsibilities. If there is any evidence or reason to believe there are physical contaminants in a food product that may cause illness or injury to consumers, government agencies, reject the food product from sale in the market or request food recalls.

Huge economic losses to businesses may occur when a physical hazard is discovered.

## Causes of Physical Contamination

Table: Sources of physical contaminants in foods.

| Sources | Examples OF Contaminants |
|---------|--------------------------|
| Field | Rock/ stones/sand, asphalt, metals/bullets, concrete particles, bones, wood fragments, and thorns. |

| Processing | Glass, Ceramic/Shards, metal fragments, staples, blades, clips, needles, keys, screws, magnet fragments, washers, bolt, bolts, screening, plastic, grease/lubricants, rubber, insulation/seal materials, nail polish, jewelry, coins, pieces of gloves, finger cots, bandages, cigarette butts, gum, bones, pits, fruit stones, nut & animal shells, medications/ tablets/capsules, wood, pens, and pencils. |
|---|---|
| Storage and distribution | Metal, plastic and wood fragments. |

Physical contaminants in food could come from either external sources, such as metal fragments, or internal sources, such as bone particles and pits. They can be introduced into food products accidentally during harvesting or at any point during processing due to poor procedural practices anywhere in the food chain, including manufacturing, storage, transportation, or retail. The so-called Dirty Dozen, the 12 most common foreign material contaminants in food, are glass, wood, stones, metal, jewelry, insects/filth, insulation, bone, plastic, personal effects, bullets/BB shot, and needles.

## Investigation and Identification of Physical Contaminants

Food companies work hard to keep their products free of contaminants. Investigation and control of physical contaminants in food should be conducted throughout the whole processing chain or in food testing laboratories. With accurate and timely information, a thorough investigation can be carried out in testing laboratories in a cost-effective and efficient manner. It is essential to have a professional investigation team with appropriate resources and equipment to help food company quality assurance staff troubleshoot consumer complaints and answer questions as to what the contaminants and their sources are. It is often necessary to apply integrated, multidimensional approaches for complicated investigations.

Comprehensive investigation can demand microscopy-based examinations plus chemical techniques, on-site examinations, Fourier transform-infrared (FTIR) analysis, and other techniques. The investigation processes and screening procedures depend on the particular physical contaminants and their sources. The procedures can be combined or modified methods found from the following: AOAC International, American Spice Trade Association, FDA's Macroanalytical Procedures Manual, FDA's Laboratory Information Bulletins, USDA's foreign matter identification documents, the United States Pharmacopeia, and other compendious sources.

In general, special investigation procedures include:

- Inspect and target suspected sources of physical contaminants.

- Identify the foreign matter.

- Determine or evaluate the root cause or sources.

These procedures consist of eight steps:

- Target contaminants: In many cases, it is necessary to select a suitable investigational procedure, including sample inspection, preparation, and identification of target contaminants. The sources of contamination are diverse, whether individual or related, or even unknown. Often, little is known about the contaminants, how many there might be, what size, what their regulatory status might be, or whether they might be in a food mixture.

Preexamination steps allow judgments to be made as to whether the targets can be separated by size, shape, mass or magnetic properties, the type of samples and contaminants (e.g., organic or inorganic), amount, circumstances of contamination, and levels. It is normally required to conduct resampling, inspection, macroscopic examination, extraction, filtration, floating, sieving, burning, dyeing, and further examination using X-ray, metal detectors/magnets, and other screening or targeting technologies. An example might be to use magnets to gather and identify ferrous metal particles from liquid samples.

- Identify contaminants: Once the suspected foreign matter screening procedures are carried out using stereo or dissecting microscopic examinations as a starting point, one can obtain detailed evidence, identifying the morphology and deciding what methods of analysis should be applied. For example, if a complainant believes that pieces of glass were observed by the naked eye in a food, it may be that the material consists of rocks, salt, sugar, plastics, minerals, struvite, or tartrate crystals. If needed, a compound microscope, bright-field/dark-field microscope, polarized microscope, or scanning electron microscope could be applied to reveal more details. Further tests are determined based on the results of microscopic examinations. Selection of such analytical strategies may require a combination of techniques or the development of multidisciplinary approaches, depending on contaminant conditions and the goals of the investigation.

- Conduct physical property tests: A polarized microscope is used to display birefringent properties from some materials, such as synthetic polymers. Spectroscopic techniques can reveal specific functional groups of a chemical material. For example, different plastics may be identified by FTIR analysis. Physical properties can be classified by many characteristics and features, such as size, shape, thickness, magnetic characteristics, solubility, buoyancy, elasticity, flexibility, flammability, temperature resistance, etc.

- Perform a chemical examination: Chemical analysis, including an elemental analysis, can reveal characteristic features that enable an understanding of chemical properties. Histochemical staining techniques are useful to test the chemical and physical properties of the contaminants. For instance, chemical reactions can be used for determination of lignin characteristics and enzymatic reactions.

- Confirm: In many cases, no single method is 100 percent guaranteed to complete an investigation and identification. Further testing may be required to validate the findings or disprove them. For example, analysis by atomic absorption spectroscopy or other elemental analysis techniques reveals different types of metals. Examination of the combustion qualities of a sample can be used to find and quantitate foreign ferrous metal particles. Protein quantitative tests can confirm the presence of animal matter.

- Compare: Building a reference library is necessary for a forensics laboratory. Identification relies on the availability of good reference library texts and official methods containing authentic reference materials as well as spectral databases to obtain definitive confirmation of the contaminants.

- Evaluate the root cause: Whether a contaminant went through a specific processing step and was introduced into the product prior to or after packaging, potential sources could be uncovered through a prudent review of all test results and existing factors. If a piece of glass was confirmed, the following question will be raised: Is it more likely to be from a lightbulb, bottle, window glass, or drinking glass? This evaluation can be done to obtain more detailed information and evidence from the contaminant's size, shape, mass, and characteristic features, especially compared with authentic reference materials. Any reference samples provided by clients are helpful to address the root cause.

- Prepare a comprehensive report: After the investigation and identification are complete, a comprehensive report should be prepared, containing a summary of the project goals, sample information, test methods, imaging evidence, findings, evaluations, and/or suggestions.

## Chemical Contamination

Chemical contamination occurs when food comes into contact with chemicals and can lead to chemical food poisoning. Chemical contamination is a global food safety issue. There are many potentially toxic substances in the environment which may contaminate foods consumed by people. They include inorganic and organic substances and may originate from a wide range of sources.

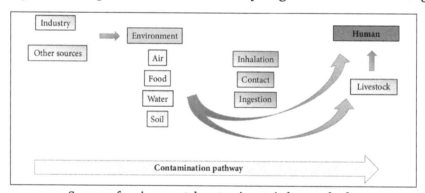

Sources of environmental contaminants in human foods.

In certain instances, the source of contaminants may be the environment. This is the case for metals such as lead and mercury, dioxins, and polychlorinated biphenyls (PCBs). Agricultural use of pesticides may lead to food contamination. Similarly, drugs used in both people and animals may contaminate waterways and pose a health risk to consumers. Additionally, food packaging methods may be a source of contamination, so-called "migrants" leaching from packing materials. These contaminants may cause acute or chronic toxic effects. Toxicity may relate to the route of exposure and dose, and personal characteristics such as age and health condition may affect the individual's susceptibility.

Due to the nature of contamination, some food products may be more contaminated than others. This may be due to several factors such as varying exposure to pesticides, differences in plant uptake mechanisms from the environment, or contaminants from food packaging. Dietary make-up will affect an individual's exposure to these contaminants. For example, nursing neonates have a high intake of contaminants that are excreted in breast milk. Exposure at different life stages may result in different toxic effects as well. For example, prenatal exposure to persistent organic pollutants has been linked to an increase in childhood obesity and increased blood pressure.

For many food items—including vegetables, fish, and other seafood—human health risk assessment data is available after analysis of available foods. Urban farms and gardens may pose additional risks due to contaminants such as metals. Furthermore, drinking water may become contaminated. Xenoestrogenic compounds have even been detected in rainwater. Water contamination may also result in pollution of marine biota, affecting suitability for consumption of seafood. Consequently individuals with high consumption of seafood will intake higher levels of such contaminants.

For most contaminants, there is no completely safe dose level. However, for many, acceptable levels have been calculated—levels below which signs of toxicity should not be evident. Toxic effects seen depend on the contaminant in question, the dose received, and the individual. For example, many contaminants have been linked to an increased risk of cancer. Skin cancer has been associated with long-term exposure to drinking water contaminated by arsenic, gastric cancer with lead contamination, and liver cancer with consumption of grain contaminated by mercury. Our understanding of the health risks from combined exposures to more than one contaminant and the means by which we can assess such interactions is lacking.

Monitoring programmes are in place both nationally and globally to monitor such contamination in order to assess food safety. However, it is important to note that such monitoring cannot completely preclude supply of contaminated food to consumers. The role of such programmes is to check that food and water contamination levels are below those deemed "unsafe." To this end, many governmental and nongovernmental organizations strive through risk assessments to ascertain what levels of contamination are acceptable for products destined for human consumption. In addition, national and international policies are in place to reduce contamination. For example, under the Stockholm Convention on Persistent Organic Pollutants, production and use of such substances are eliminated or restricted. This international treaty came into force in 2004 and currently has 152 signatories from 182 parties. The Codex Alimentarius describes international food standards, setting permitted maximum levels (ML) for contaminants in foods based on risk assessment and scientific evidence. The Codex Committee on Contaminants in Food (CCCF) is a global forum, but it can be difficult to compromise national legislations and harmonize global standards. Lists of contaminants also undergo risk assessment by the Joint FAO/WHO Expert Committee on Food Additives. Recommendations are made for standards such as provisional maximum tolerable daily intake (PMTDI) or provisional tolerable weekly intake (PTWI). These are usually calculated based on chronic toxicity data, and thus it may also be useful to consider acute reference doses (ARfDs). The Codex Committee on Pesticide Residues (CCPR) has established maximum residue limits (MRLs) for over 5,000 pesticide residues. This committee also considers reports from the FAO/WHO Meeting on Pesticide Residues (JMPR), which estimates MRLs and acceptable daily intakes (ADIs) for people.

## Sources of Contaminants from the Environment to Food and Water

It is useful to consider the sources of contaminants in order to understand their pathway into food and water sources for consumption. Factors such as soil properties, activities by people, and point sources affect the accumulation of metals in the environment. For example, mining may result in release of substances such as arsenic and mercury. Once in the environment, these substances may contaminate food and water and result in human health hazards, with toxic effects varying depending on the contaminant(s) ingested.

## Metals and Metalloids

Metals and metalloids in the environment have various sources. One source of mercury and lead is artisanal gold mining. For example, in the gold mining area of Tongguan, Shaanxi, China, concentrations of these metals in locally produced grains and vegetables exceeded governmental tolerance limits and posed a potential health risk to people from consumption. Lead and cadmium from an iron mine in Morocco resulted in concentrations of cadmium in livestock organs higher than acceptable limits. Likewise, in Spain, sheep near a mine were found to have lead contamination, with levels in 87.5% liver samples above European Union Maximum Residue Levels (MRL).

Industrial regions often have extensive environmental contamination by metals. In Romania, lead, cadmium, copper, and zinc contaminated crops, exceeding maximum acceptable levels in some samples. In China, cadmium from a zinc smelter contaminated leaf and root vegetables particularly. Arsenic, selenium, lead, and other metal and metalloid contaminants were found near a coking plant in China, contaminating soil and food, and detected in blood samples from children. In that case, ingestion of food was determined to be the major exposure pathway for local children. In Belgium, cadmium was detected in locally produced food items grown near nonferrous metal plants. Thallium from a steel plant in south China was found to contaminate soil and thence vegetables, exceeding German standards for the maximum permissible level and showing hyper accumulation in plants such as leaf lettuce, chard, and pak choi.

Many fruits and vegetables have been shown to be contaminated by metals. For example, cadmium in soil was detected in navel oranges in China and lead and cadmium in soybeans in Argentina. Also in China, various metals were detected in edible seeds, with levels of copper sufficiently high to show an increased health risk to people consuming them. On the contrary, contamination levels of mercury in rice samples from a city in eastern China were below levels likely to affect human health. In the global arena, methylmercury has been detected in fish and other seafood around the world. Fish tissues from Turkey were shown to be contaminated with copper, iron, zinc, and manganese. Various metals have also been detected in fish from Sicily, with some concentrations exceeding European regulation limits. In Asia, food species of turtles have been shown to contain mercury.

With regard to water, endemic arsenism from contaminated drinking water has been reported in China. Monitoring has detected nickel in drinking water in New South Wales, Australia, but levels do not appear to pose any health risk for the local population.

Further evidence of potential health risks to people from metals are surveys of human samples. Mercury and monomethylmercury were detected in human hair samples from French Guiana, associated with a diet rich in fish, with 57% of people tested having mercury levels higher than the WHO safety limit. In Spain, mercury, lead, and cadmium have also been detected in human milk samples, with increased levels of lead associated with higher consumption of potatoes.

## Polycyclic Aromatic Hydrocarbons

Polycyclic aromatic hydrocarbons (PAHs) primarily occur after organic matter undergoes incomplete combustion or pyrolysis, or from industrial processes. Food contamination comes from the environment, industry, or home cooking (such as when using biomass fuels). These compounds appear to be genotoxic and carcinogenic. Oil spills from transporter ships in the ocean are all too common and will result in contamination of seafood. Besides the petroleum-related polycyclic aromatic hydrocarbon (PAH) compounds, chemical dispersants are often used to mitigate effects of oil in the ocean. After the BP Deepwater Horizon oil spill in Louisiana, USA, in 2010, the Federal government responded to seafood safety concerns by instigating protocols for sampling and analysis of food to determine its safety. Lessons learned after this scenario included recognition of the need to improve risk assessments to adequately protect vulnerable populations, including pregnant women.

## Industrial Chemicals

Persistent organic pollutants (POPs) are synthetic organic chemicals; some are used in industry, some as pesticides, and some are by-products from industry or combustion. They include pesticides like aldrin, chlordane and DDT, industrial chemicals like PCBs and HCBs, and unintended by-products like dibenzodioxins and dibenzofurans. They persist in the environment, are distributed globally in air and ocean currents, and accumulate in animals in the food chain (including in humans). Their side effects depend on the chemical and the contaminated species; for example, they may have effects on reproductive or immune systems, or increase cancer risks.

Chlorpyrifos is an organophosphate pesticide that affects vision and causes other neurological toxic effects in humans. It has been detected in dietary samples, and foods have been shown to be responsible for approximately 13% of daily exposure to this chemical. Organochlorine pesticides such as DDT have been used in agriculture and vector-transmitted disease control for decades, though their use now is restricted due to known persistence in the environment and toxic effects such as neurological dysfunction and endocrine disruption. Pyrethroids such as permethrin and deltamethrin are widely used for control of vector insects and aircraft disinfection, as they are relatively safe for people. However, their use near foods can result in contamination and studies are ongoing to reduce potential toxic effects. Although neonicotinoids are widespread in the environment and contaminate consumable items, their toxic effects are still not yet well understood.

Polychlorinated biphenyls (PCBs) have a variety of uses in industry, including in transformers, as heat exchange fluids or paint additives, or in plastics. Ingestion of PCB residue-contaminated food—especially meat, fish, and poultry—is the main source for people, with ready absorption from the gastrointestinal tract. Contaminated breast milk is a potential source for nursing infants. Chloracne is reported after extensive exposure to PCBs, but immune and carcinogenic effects may also result.

Polybrominated and polychlorinated compounds may originate from anthropogenic and natural sources. They have many uses such as flame retardants and dielectric/coolant fluids in electrical apparatus. Toxic effects include endocrine disruption, neurotoxicity, and cancer. Polybrominated diphenyl ethers (PBDEs) and polychlorinated biphenyls (PCBs) have been detected in human milk in China. This is a particular concern due to the high susceptibility of nursing infants to toxic effects. According to a study in Germany, dietary exposure is the most significant pathway for PB-DEs in people. In particular, seafood has been cited as a major contributor.

Perfluorinated compounds (PFCs) are synthetic chemicals with friction-resistant properties that make them useful in many materials and industries. Toxic effects include endocrine and immune system disruption and developmental problems. Some precursors or metabolic intermediates for perfluoroalkyl and polyfluoroalkyl substances (PFASs) are toxic, for example, estrogen-like activities. The PFAS group includes perfluorooctane sulfonic acid (PFOS) and perfluorooctanoic acid (PFOA); these have been detected in many food sources including seafood in China and Germany. Drinking water and food are the main sources of exposure to PFOS and PFOA, although levels are usually low.

Acrylamide occurs in many foods—generally associated with high heat cooking processes (e.g., in breads and baked or fried potatoes)—and is also manufactured for commercial and industrial uses (such as in paper and dye production, in wastewater treatment, and as a chemical grouting agent). The IARC has classified acrylamide as a probable human carcinogen, placed in group 2A since 1994.

## Pharmaceuticals and Personal Care Products

The term pharmaceuticals and personal care products (PPCPs) includes a wide range of substances that may enter the environment and thence food or water sources. Antimicrobials and other drugs may originate from use in both humans and animals. For example, swine waste containing antimicrobials may contaminate both water and food. Aside from the very real threat of increased antimicrobial resistance through exposure to extraneous sources of these chemicals, it has also been shown that many drugs have other side effects including endocrine disruption. In some circumstances, the medicinal products themselves may be contaminated, for example, in many herbal products.

## Radioactive Elements

Most radioactive elements did not exist naturally, and soil contamination with such material has only become a problem since nuclear weapons and reactors have been developed.

After tsunami damage affected the Fukushima nuclear plant in Japan in 2011, monitoring of food and water samples detected contamination above provisional regulation values and restrictions were put in place. Radionucleotides have also been detected in seafood in India, various foods in the Balkans, and food and drinking water in Switzerland. Risk assessments are conducted to ensure that levels remain within acceptable limits. Furthermore, experimental models are undertaken to assess safety in ingestion pathways, considering several different food intakes. In the US, there is an FDA rule pertaining to uranium, radium, alpha particle, beta particle, and photon radioactivity in bottled water.

## Electronic Waste

Modern society has become encumbered with many electrical devices, and electronic waste (or e-waste) has become a major problem. Inappropriate processing, for example, incomplete combustion, of such products releases a variety of pollutants covered above, including PBDEs, dioxins/furans (PCDD/Fs), PAHs, PCBs, and metals/metalloids. In addition, contamination from such devices can enter drinking water and food.

## Plastics

In recent times, we rely more and more on packaging materials—in particular plastics—to transport and help preserve food. These materials are not inert and may themselves contaminate food and drinks as multiple chemicals are released into foods and beverages from food contact materials. These are termed "migrants" and include such chemicals as phthalate plasticizers which have been detected in bottled water. Factors such as higher storage temperatures and prolonged contact time with the packaging were linked to higher levels of contamination, but a health risk assessment showed that the risk for consumers was low.

## Nanoparticles

Another recent development is that of nanoparticles. These have one dimension less than $1 \times 10{-7}$ m, and engineered nanoparticles have been used in a wide range of products, such as paints, cosmetics, and pesticides. Pathways and effects of these in biota are as yet unclear, but they have been shown to travel in the food chain. Nanosized materials have been detected in foods such as wheat-based products.

## Risk Assessment and Monitoring

The possible contaminants in food can be linked to a variety of toxic effects. Any adverse effects seen depend on multiple factors, including whether exposure is acute or chronic, the dose received, the route of exposure, and details of the individual person such as age and health. As an example, lead toxicity affects almost all organs, but the most severely affected is the nervous system. In adults, long-term exposure results in reduced cognitive performance. More severe signs such as learning difficulties and behavioural problems are seen in infants and young children as they are more sensitive during this phase of neurodevelopment. High levels of contamination with lead may also cause kidney damage; chronic exposure may cause anaemia and hypertension, and reduced fertility in males. In pregnant women, high blood lead levels are associated with premature birth or babies with a low birth weight, and this risk is increased in emaciated women. On an individual level, blood sampling is a quick and easy method of assessing circulating levels of lead and can be used to indicate recent or current exposure. However, this does not account for lead stored elsewhere in the body, particularly in bones. X-ray fluorescence can measure whole-body lead in bones, and x-rays may show lead-containing foreign materials. Treatment of clinical cases is by using chelating agents, which will reduce blood lead levels, yet neurological effects may remain.

On the other hand, at a community level, it may be more important to identify contaminated sites and assess health risks to the general population and thereafter aim to reduce or remove exposure to contaminants such as lead. Thus, monitoring plays a vital role in food safety. Such monitoring has identified contamination of many foods. In order to monitor effectively, samples should be analysed from a variety of sources: human samples to detect levels after exposure, diverse foods from the total diet and drinking water sources, and also the environment itself (to identify the source of food contamination). Samples from people frequently include blood, urine, feces, breast milk, hair, and/or semen. Human biomonitoring is notably useful to facilitate risk assessment. A combination of environmental monitoring and biomonitoring may identify risk factors, such as detection of higher levels of cadmium in umbilical cord blood from mothers consuming more than two portions of fish each week. In the case of metals, environmental sampling has shown hotspots of contamination around mining (such as gold, lead, and zinc), electronic waste sites, and industrial areas. Contamination in soils at these sites has been linked to bioaccumulation in agricultural crops and associated increase in human health risk.

Examples of indirect monitoring methods for contaminants in the environment and food include measurement of biomarkers such as proteomics in oysters contaminated with mercury, transcriptome effects in the hepatopancreas of clams, or mutagenicity of seawater in seafood farms associated with PAHs and PCBs. High throughput and ultrasensitive screening using nanoparticles has also been utilized for detection of environmental pollutants. Moving forward, testing of chemicals to evaluate potential toxicities before registration and authorised use in the environment may employ tools and concepts such as biomonitoring equivalents and threshold of toxicologic concern, alongside generic and physiologically-based toxicokinetic models. Since 2006, the European Commission has implemented new legislation, called REACH (EC 1907/2006), to identify properties—including toxicities—of chemicals and thus better protect human health and the environment. Other similar legislation exists elsewhere in the world; for example, the Environmental Protection Agency runs a registration process for pesticides to comply with federal laws in the US.

Once sources of contaminants have been identified, it is vital to minimize contamination of food. For this purpose, regulations are in place at both national and international levels to restrict contaminated food entering the human food chain. In some cases, legislation exists to assess levels of food contamination. For example, the Marine Strategy Framework Directive in Spain monitors for contaminants in edible tissues of seafood destined for human consumption, assessing levels against established EU standards for food safety. The German Federal Environment Agency monitors both the environment—using the German Environmental Survey (GerES)—and human biomonitoring—using the German Environmental Specimen Bank (ESB). Amongst others, these have, respectively, been used to detect lead in drinking water and exposure to phthalates and bisphenol A. National monitoring systems may cooperate at an international level. To maintain and improve food safety globally, the Codex Alimentarius contains a set of international food standards, guidelines, and codes of practice. These are based on science from risk assessment bodies or organized by consultations with FAO and WHO. These are voluntary but often form the basis of national legislation.

Food standards and legislation focus on individual food products. To understand the combined risk that someone has from one or many chemicals, a complete dietary risk assessment can be conducted to assess the total potential risk of a typical diet. For example, Zhou et al. assessed the levels of organochlorine pesticides (OCPs) in a total diet from China. The study found that aquatic foods, meats, and cereals were the major foods contributing to contamination of the diet with these chemicals. Multilevel risk assessment can also be used to identify critical points in contamination sources. For example, a study of metals in soil and food in Taiwan identified more than 600 metal-contaminated sites over a period of two decades which could then be targeted for remediation efforts.

# Remediation

Once sources of contamination have been identified, it is possible to consider how best to improve food safety through various methods. Methods of remediation vary depending on the type of contaminants present and in which environment. These can be expensive on a large scale. Remediation may focus on reducing contaminants in the environment overall or reducing concentrations in foods specifically.

A common method used to reduce environmental exposure to contaminants is soil remediation. One simple method is to remove contaminated topsoil, which typically contains higher levels of contaminants than subsoil, from agricultural areas. Alternatively, soil turnover and mixing in situ may be sufficient to dilute contaminant, such as metals, concentrations to an acceptable level. Thermal treatment or landfill can also be used to remediate a site. Different soil properties can affect contaminant levels. For example, metal (cadmium, mercury, and chromium) accumulation in flowering Chinese cabbage was shown to be controlled by total metal concentrations in soil and available calcium. It is well known that soil science can be used to improve food quality and quantity. It can similarly be used to reduce contamination of crops. The predominant congener of technical DDT, p,p'-DDT, is susceptible to microbial metabolism and rarely accumulates in aerobic soils. Long-term gardening has been shown to result in lower levels of PAHs, possibly due to PAH degradation by enhanced microbial activity, and/or dilution. Microbial bioremediation may also be used to reduce levels of metal contamination of soils in an environmentally-friendly manner.

Different forms of phytoremediation may be used to either remove contamination from soils or to reduce contamination of plants. If the plants are crops for consumption, reduced uptake is beneficial. One example of phytoremediation is selection of plants to specifically remove contaminants from agricultural land, such as using black nightshade (Solanum nigrum L.) for removal of thallium from soil. A study by Yu et al. on cadmium-contaminated agricultural land showed differential accumulation of cadmium in two oilseed rape cultivars. Interestingly, the study also showed increased uptake of cadmium in rice crops planted after the oilseed rape harvest, with contamination of rice higher compared to a crop after a fallow period. Another mechanism of plants which can be used advantageously is that of reduced accumulation of unwanted chemicals in certain cultivars or altered plant hybrids—for example in Chinese kale—and these can be selected to produce safer food.

Crop management techniques can affect contamination of plants. Use of slow-release nitrogen fertilizers can reduce cadmium levels in plants such as pak choi, as the plants appear to have stronger tolerance to the metal and a lower efficiency of translocation to edible plant parts compared to those grown using typical fertilizers. Contaminated water used to flood paddy fields is a huge problem in countries that rely on rice crops. Water management—such as drying the paddy field for a period of days between late tillering and young ear differentiation stages—has been shown to reduce cadmium and arsenic levels in rice crops of different rice species. Human health risks from medicinal products contaminating food and water for consumption may be modelled, for example, using pond aquaculture, to identify potential health risks.

Exposure to contaminants on foods prepared for consumption can also be reduced by using safer storage alternatives, such as edible films and coatings. Contamination of foods with PAHs from cooking can be greatly reduced by avoiding smoking or open fires but rather replacing them with gas stoves for cooking. Several nongovernmental organizations and charities offer gas stoves to families to help alleviate this source of food contamination, which is a risk particularly for women and children who spend more time at home.

# Cross-contamination

Cross-contamination is the transfer of harmful bacteria to food from other foods, cutting boards, utensils, etc., if they are not handled properly. This is especially true when handling raw meat, poultry, and seafood, so keep these foods and their juices away from already cooked or ready-to-eat foods and fresh produce.

However, it is not just bacteria that gets carried from one place to another—it could also be a virus or a toxin of some kind, or even a cleaning product. But whatever it is, if it comes into contact with someone's food, it's considered cross-contamination. And if they eat the food and it makes them sick, it is called food poisoning. As a home cook, though, there are quite a few steps you can take and habits you can build to help reduce the likelihood of cross-contamination in your kitchen.

Since dangerous bacteria are killed by high heat, the risk of cross-contamination is highest with food that doesn't need to be cooked. That's why outbreaks of salmonella poisoning are increasingly found to be linked to foods like sprouts and bagged salads, foods you might think of as innocuous or "safe" but are risky because they customarily aren't cooked.

Cross-contamination can happen on a very large scale because of equipment at processing facilities not being cleaned properly, for instance, or any of the other numerous ways your food can be mishandled as it makes its way to your kitchen. This is why, from time to time, there are outbreaks of food poisoning, product recalls, restaurant closures, and the like. And, unfortunately, there's not much you can do to protect yourself at that level, other than keeping track of the news and using good sense in deciding which ingredients to purchase and where to eat out.

When it comes to cross-contamination in the home, in nearly all cases, it is going to be caused either by your kitchen knife, your cutting board, or your hands (and once it's on your hands, it's on everything else as well). The knife and cutting board really are the major culprits, though, since almost everything touches your cutting board and the knife—cutting up food on a cutting board is, after all, a big part of cooking.

When handling foods, it is important to Be Smart, Keep Foods Apart — Don't Cross-Contaminate. By following these simple steps, you can prevent cross-contamination and reduce the risk of foodborne illness.

## When Shopping

Separate raw meat, poultry, and seafood from other foods in your grocery-shopping cart. Place these foods in plastic bags to prevent their juices from dripping onto other foods. It is also best to separate these foods from other foods at check out and in your grocery bags.

## When Refrigerating Food

- Place raw meat, poultry, and seafood in containers or sealed plastic bags to prevent their juices from dripping onto other foods. Raw juices often contain harmful bacteria.

- Store eggs in their original carton and refrigerate as soon as possible.

## When Preparing Food

Wash hands and surfaces often. Harmful bacteria can spread throughout the kitchen and get onto cutting boards, utensils, and counter tops. To prevent this:

- Wash hands with soap and warm water for 20 seconds before and after handling food, and after using the bathroom, changing diapers; or handling pets.

- Use hot, soapy water and paper towels or clean clothes to wipe up kitchen surfaces or spills. Wash cloths often in the hot cycle of your washing machine.

- Wash cutting boards, dishes, and counter tops with hot, soapy water after preparing each food item and before you go on to the next item.

- A solution of 1 tablespoon of unscented, liquid chlorine bleach per gallon of water may be used to sanitize surfaces and utensils.

## Cutting Boards

- Always use a clean cutting board.

- If possible, use one cutting board for fresh produce and a separate one for raw meat, poultry, and seafood.

- Once cutting boards become excessively worn or develop hard-to-clean grooves, you should replace them.

## Marinating Food

- Always marinate food in the refrigerator, not on the counter.

- Sauce that is used to marinate raw meat, poultry, or seafood should not be used on cooked foods, unless it is boiled just before using.

## When Serving Food

- Always use a clean plate.

- Never place cooked food back on the same plate or cutting board that previously held raw food.

## When Storing Leftovers

Refrigerate or freeze leftovers within 2 hours or sooner in clean, shallow, covered containers to prevent harmful bacteria from multiplying.

# Shelf Life of Food

Shelf life is the period of time that food can be kept before it starts to deteriorate and begins from the time the food is prepared or manufactured.

Its length is dependent on many factors including:

- The types of ingredients,

- Manufacturing process,

- Type of packaging and how the food is stored.

Shelf life it is indicated by labeling the product with a date mark.

Controlling the pathogen content (safety) of foods should be achieved by using a Hazard Analysis Critical Control Point (HACCP) system.

Predictive modeling or challenge testing can be used to assess pathogen growth. Food safety and product shelf life are inextricably linked.

During the shelf life of a food it should:

- Remain safe to eat.

- Keep its appearance, odor, texture and flavor.

- Meet any nutritional claims provided on the label.

The EU Standards Code defines composition and labeling requirements for all food sold in EU and all over the world.

The shelf life is defined in Standard s which requires that any packaged food with a shelf life of less than two years be labeled with a date mark.

The Code requires food to be safe up to, and including, the date marked.

One of the following options must be used:

- A "Use by" date: This is used for highly perishable foods that will present a safety risk if consumed after this date. A food must not be sold if it is past its "Use by" date, nor should it be consumed.

- A "Best before" date: This is used for foods other than those specified above. It is not illegal to sell food that has reached its "Best before" date.

- "Baked on" and "Baked for" date marks can be used on bread products with a shelf life of less than 7 days. The "Baked for" date must be no later than 12 hours after the bread was baked.

What does the date mark look like? The words "Use by", "Best before", or "Baked on" must be followed by a date or a reference to where on the package the date is located.

The date must have:

- At least the day and the month for products with a shelf life of up to three months e.g. best before 24 March.

- At least the month and the year for products with a shelf life over three months e.g. June 2016.

The dates must be expressed numerically and chronologically (day month year) but the month can be expressed in letters. These must be "not coded".

"Packed on" dates or packer's codes can be used but only in addition to the date marks described above.

The Code also states:

- Specific storage instructions must be included on the label where these are necessary to ensure the food will keep for the specified period indicated by the date marking.

- Storage conditions must be achievable in the distribution and retail systems and in the home.

- The seller must store the food according to stated storage instructions.

- Consideration also needs to be given to providing directions for use and storage after opening.

Anyone who packages and sells food that is required to be date marked is legally responsible for calculating how long their product can reasonably be expected to keep, without any appreciable change in quality. The food label is required to detail the shelf life and the storage instructions to meet that shelf life.

For shelf life determination, the evaluator is required to understand basic food science and technology including food processing, food analysis, food packaging, and statistical techniques. Shelf life studies must be carried out only when foods are correctly processed, packed, and stored, ready for purchase and consumption. The end of shelf life can be determined from (1) relevant food legislation; (2) guidelines given by enforcement authorities or agencies; (3) guides provided by independent professional bodies such as IFT; (4) current industrial best practice; (5) self-imposed end-point assessment; and (6) market information.

## Factors Affecting the Shelf Life Test

## Understand the Product

The evaluators should ensure that they understand the product very well. In general, the food product can be classified into three types as follows: (1) Highly perishable foods (milk, fresh meat, fresh fruits, and vegetables) – These are very short-shelf life products that are subject to microbiological and/or enzymatic deterioration. Measurements are taken every day in order to determine shelf life. (2) Semiperishable foods (pasteurized milk, smoked meats, cheeses, and some bakery products) – These are short-to-medium shelf life products and may contain natural inhibitors or have received minimal preservative treatment Measurements are made every week in order to determine shelf life. (3) Highly stable foods (dried food, canned food, and frozen food) – these are medium-to-long shelf life products that have received a thermal process or are maintained in specific conditions. Measurements are made every week or monthly in order to determine shelf life.

## Understand the Factors affecting Product Quality

Many factors can influence shelf life and can be categorized into compositional and environmental factors. Compositional factors are the properties of the final product including food composition; water activity (aw); pH value; total acidity; type of acid; redox potential (Eh); available oxygen, nutrients, natural microflora, and surviving microbiological counts; natural biochemistry of the product formulation (enzymes, chemical reactants); use of preservatives in product formulation (e.g., salt); and concentration of reactant, inhibitor, and catalyst.

For environmental factors, they are those factors the final product encounters as it moves through the food chain including time–temperature profile during processing; pressure in the headspace; temperature control during storage and distribution; relative humidity (RH) during processing, storage, and distribution; exposure to light (UV and IR) during processing, storage, and distribution; environmental microbial counts during processing, storage, and distribution; atmospheric composition within packaging; subsequent heat treatment (e.g., reheating or cooking before consumption); and distributor, retailer, and consumer handling.

## Identify the Critical Quality based on several Guidelines

These guidelines include (1) government law – the critical quality is mainly for microbial safety; (2) customer standard – this may be higher than the government standard; (3) competitors – the critical quality can be related to a competitor's product; and (4) consumers – they provide the best judgment of the critical quality of each food.

## Understand the Concerted Series

These series of biochemical/physicochemical reactions are required to insightfully understand and identify mechanisms responsible for spoilage or loss of desirable characteristics. Several reactions involve food deterioration such as microbiological spoilage, chemical and enzymatic activity including rancidity, browning reactions, and moisture and/or other vapor migration.

## Types of Shelf Life Tests and Design

The shelf life test can be divided into three types including the following:

### Static Tests

Product stored under a given set of environmental conditions. This test requires a long time to observe changes and is expensive. It gives no information on the effects of stress and comes the closest to distribution conditions.

### Accelerated Tests

Product stored under a range of environmental conditions (usually temperature or relative humidity). The conditions of this test are selected to cover the expected range encountered and can be achieved in a relatively short period of time. It also provides kinetic data, and the test conditions should not alter the normal anticipated path affecting shelf life. The results must be interpreted with care.

## Use/Abuse Tests

Product cycled through environmental variables. The test is used to assess the product and package as a unit. These tests use cycles of variables that are equal to or beyond that expected under actual conditions. It is often used to determine the effects of transport.

## Storage and Sampling Design

Design of the shelf life test is very important. There are several relevant criteria for shelf life testing. The factor has enough effect on the quality changes, and the critical parameter is directly related to quality and consumer acceptance. In addition, the parameter is easy to determine with simple and practical design. There are enough samples, and the quality of sample can be controlled. The evaluator should concern about the method of measurement: it is standard and appropriate. This is relevant to the cost of testing. Homogeneity of the sample such as yoghurt with fruit pieces should be prepared very well to make sure that the sample represents the whole product.

For microbial safety consideration, it is very critical. The sample should not be tested for other qualities (especially sensory tests) prior to microbiological testing results. For frozen product, it is noticed that biochemical changes in food can occur during frozen storage. Therefore, the relationship of several parameters can be related and should be considered.

For accelerated test involved with temperature, the temperature differences can vary from 5 to 10 °C, and extremely high storage temperatures should be avoided. The sample during storage tests should include around six to eight points of sampling time. The quality changes of the product should be 30–50% of the original to represent an accurate trend of deterioration. In general, product sampling during storage tests can be divided into three types:

- Basic Design Sampling: The sample will be collected for product quality assessment following the sampling plan, for example, once a week until the end of shelf life analysis. The advantage of this design is that the frequency of sampling can be increased or decreased as appropriate. However, if the sample would be tested for sensory panels, especially trained panels, the cost of this design will be high due to repeated training of panels before each test.

- Reverse Design Sampling: The sample will be collected following the sampling plan; however, the sample will be maintained under controlled conditions. The controlled condition ensures that the sample quality is quite stable, such as freezing or refrigeration. The sample will be assessed after the completion of all samplings at the same time. The advantage of this design is the lower cost for sensory testing. However, a problem may arise if the sample changes are faster or later than expected.

- Semireverse Design Sampling: This is another option for sampling and is a combination of the basic and reverse sampling. The sample may be collected for testing after two to three rounds of sampling or in the middle of the sampling plan to ensure that the product quality changes are within the expected range of deterioration.

## Storage Test and Trial Conditions

The guidelines for shelf life testing conditions are as follows:

## Storage Conditions

The sample should be stored in several conditions including optimum conditions, typical or average conditions, and worst-case conditions.

## Commonly used for Fixed-storage Conditions

- Frozen: 18 °C or lower (RH is usually close to 100%).

- Chilled: 0–5 °C, with a maximum of 8°C (RH is usually very high).

- Temperate: 25 °C, 75% RH l Tropical: 38°C, 90% RH.

- Control: Optimum conditions for each product.

## Samples for Storage Trials

Number of samples should be concerned. Size and packaging of samples should be the same and close to real conditions.

## Sampling Schedule

The sampling plan is depended on the typical shelf life: (1) Short-shelf life products: Up to 1 week (e.g., ready meals), samples can be taken off daily for evaluation. (2) Medium-shelf life products: Up to 3 weeks (e.g., some ambient cakes and pastry), samples can be taken off on days 0, 7, 14, 19, 21, and 25. (3) Long-shelf life products: Up to 1 year (e.g., some breakfast cereals), samples can be taken off at monthly intervals or at months 0, 1, 2, 3, 6, 12, and (perhaps) 18.

## Kinetic Reactions

The simplest technique for shelf life testing is the kinetic reaction approach. To predict the shelf life, the kinetic data is used to evaluate how the deterioration process behaves as a function of time. It is the concept of quantification of the quality of food products based on reaction change. The kinetic equation may be expressed as:

$$r_A = -\frac{d[A]}{dt} = k[A]^n.$$

Following the chemical reactions, k is the kinetic constant, t is time, and n is order of reaction. The change in concentration A of a component of interest is monitored. The quality factors [A] are usually quantifiable chemical, physical, microbiological, or sensory parameters, such as the loss of a nutrient or characteristic of flavor or formation of an off-flavor. The time to reach the value of the quality index ( $A_{t_s}$ ) at a specified condition (i.e., the shelf life) $t_s$ is inversely proportional to the rate constant at these conditions.

$$t_s = \frac{f_q(A_{t_s})}{k}$$

Table: Quality function of reaction order.

| Apparent reaction order | Quality function |
|---|---|
| 0 | $A_t - A_0$ or $A_t/A_0$ |
| 1 | $\ln(A_t - A_0)$ or $\ln(A_t/A_0)$ |
| 2 | $1/A_t - 1/A_0$ |
| n (n ≠ 1) | $(1/n-1).(A_t^{1-n} - A_0^{1-n})$ |

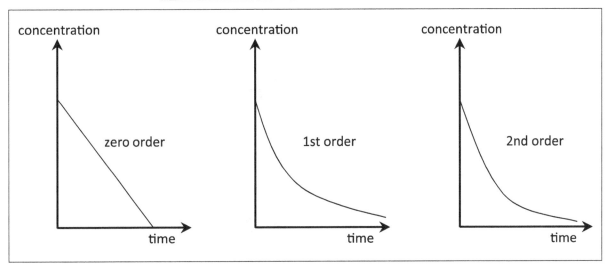

Pattern of concentration changes in different reaction orders.

The forms of the quality function of the food for an apparent zero-, first-, second- or nth-order reaction are presented in Table and Figure, which show the different patterns of the reaction orders. For zero-order reactions, the reaction rate is independent of the concentration of a reactant. First-order reactions depend on a single reactant, and the exponent value is one. For second-order reactions, the reaction rate may be proportional to one concentration squared or to the product of two concentrations. Most reactions that are responsible for shelf life loss based on a characteristic physicochemical, chemical, or microbial index include the following: zero order (e.g., frozen food overall quality, Maillard browning) and first order (e.g., vitamin loss, oxidative color loss, microbial growth), as shown in Table and Figure. Several published research has been applied to the kinetic model to describe the temperature dependence. The quality parameters can be chemical properties such as peroxide value in extra virgin olive oil; vitamin C loss in citrus juice concentrate; hydrogen ion in coffee liquids; physical property such as color loss in fresh-cut asparagus; weight loss in frozen bread dough; or sensory property such as sensory attributes in frozen shrimp.

The simplest and frequently used method to find the reaction order is the integration method. The process starts from (1) guess reaction order; (2) integrate; (3) linearize by linear regression; (4) plot experimental data in linearized form; and (5) if data fit a straight line, then guess is right, if not start again. The simple selection is higher coefficient of determination ($R_2$), and slope is reaction rate constant. Determination of reaction order has been exemplified in Example 1 as follows:

Example: Determination of reaction order.

Find the reaction order of ascorbic acid loss on multivitamin storage. The concentrations of ascorbic acid (A) at different times when stored at 40 °C are presented in Table.

Solution: Guess reaction order by applying the quality function as shown in Table. Then, plot graph to compare each order as shown in figure. From the plot in figure, the best fit is the first-order reaction.

Table: Concentrations of ascorbic acid at different times when stored at 40 °C.

| Time (days) | Ascorbic acid (mg ml$^{-1}$) |
|---|---|
| 10 | 271 |
| 20 | 109 |
| 30 | 58 |
| 40 | 30.5 |
| 50 | 18 |
| 60 | 10 |

Table: Comparison of reaction orders.

| Time (days) | Zero order (A) | First order (ln A) | Second order (1/A) |
|---|---|---|---|
| 10 | 271 | 5.602119 | 0.00369 |
| 20 | 109 | 4.691348 | 0.009174 |
| 30 | 58 | 4.060443 | 0.017241 |
| 40 | 30.5 | 3.417727 | 0.032787 |
| 50 | 18 | 2.890372 | 0.055556 |
| 60 | 10 | 2.302585 | 0.1 |
| $R^2$ | 0.7522 | 0.9916 | 0.8758 |

## Accelerated Shelf Life Simulation

Food industries require a relatively short time to obtain the necessary information for determining the shelf life of their products. For practical reasons, when the actual storage time is long, the industry usually uses accelerated test techniques that considerably shorten the process of obtaining the necessary experimental data. Accelerated shelf life simulation will refer to any method that is capable of evaluating product stability, based on data that is obtained in a significantly shorter period than the actual shelf life of the product. As aimed at shortening the time required to estimate a shelf life, the concepts of accelerated shelf life simulation include: (1) The assumption is that by storing food at a higher temperature, any adverse effect on its storage behavior and hence shelf life may become apparent in a shorter time. (2) The shelf life under normal storage conditions can be estimated by extrapolation using the data obtained from the accelerated determination.

## Steps of Accelerated Shelf Life Simulation

When the accelerated shelf life testing is performed, the compositional factors must be kept constant. For full concern, the microbial safety and quality parameters must be defined and determined as the first priority for shelf life of product. Then, key deteriorative reactions that will cause quality loss and consumer unacceptability are selected. In case of proper packaging, the cost-effective packages are used except the effect of packaging materials is concerned. The different packaging materials will be used for comparison. Otherwise, the other environmental factors, including temperature, relative humidity, light, etc., as the desired kinetically active factors for acceleration of the deterioration process are selected.

Next step, the evaluator should determine how long the product is to be held at each test temperature and determine the frequency of test time between tests at temperature. The overall number of samples that must be stored at each temperature value will be calculated.

Final step is that a kinetic study of the deterioration process at such levels of the accelerating factors is run. However, if the rate of deterioration is too fast or too slow, then the frequency of sampling can be increased or decreased as appropriate. The shelf life prediction can be predicted by constructing the shelf life plots to determine the shelf life under normal storage conditions using the extrapolating data or the kinetic model to predict shelf life at actual storage conditions.

## Arrhenius Model

The Arrhenius model is a classical model that relates the rate of a chemical reaction to the changes in temperature. This model is widely applied in several processing and storage tests as affected by temperature. The model is represented by:

$$k = k_0 \ \exp\left(-\frac{E_a}{RT}\right),$$

where $k_0$ is the rate constant, $E_a$ is the energy of activation, R is the gas constant (1.9872 cal mol$^{-1}$ K$^{-1}$ or 8.3144 J mol$^{-1}$ K$^{-1}$), and T is the absolute temperature (Kelvin, K). The Arrhenius equation can be put in standard slope-intercept form by taking the natural logarithm by:

$$
\begin{aligned}
\ln k \quad &= \ln A \quad -E_a / RT \qquad \text{or} \\
\ln k \quad &= \ln A \quad -(E_a / R) \quad \times (1/T) \\
\updownarrow \quad &\quad \updownarrow \qquad\quad \updownarrow \qquad\qquad \updownarrow \\
y \quad &= b \qquad\quad +a \qquad\qquad x
\end{aligned}
$$

The steps of the Arrhenius model for shelf life determination are as follows:

- Find the reaction order following the kinetic reaction concept.

- Follow the Arrhenius relationship.

- Plot the Arrhenius relationship.

- Fit the curve using linear regression.

- Slope of plot between ln k versus 1/T is Ea/R. For instance, Arrhenius model having been employed for shelf life prediction is demonstrated in example below.

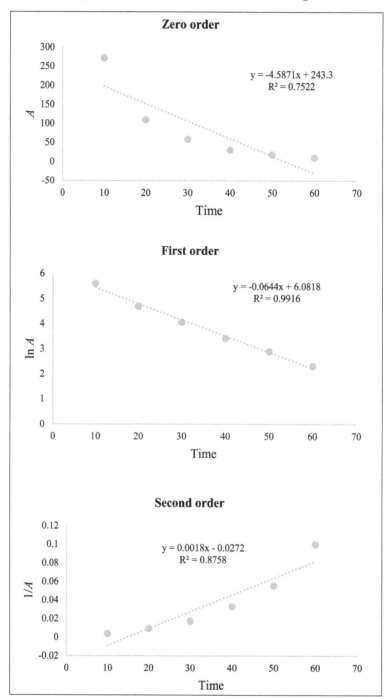

Plots of data representing quality function of reaction order.

Example: Application of the Arrhenius model for shelf life prediction.

To investigate the effect of propolis extract obtained from a domestic source in Thailand on the antioxidant properties of six mayonnaise formulas during storage. Propolis was extracted using 95% ethanol in a 1:3 (w/w) ratio for 14 days. The effects of propolis extract (0%, 0.25%, and

0.5%) and fish oil (0% and 2%) on mayonnaise stored at 5 °C, 35 °C, or 55 °C for 0, 1, 2, 3, and 4 weeks were determined. The results of acid value (AV) tests during storage as shown in Table can be described by a zero-order reaction. The correlation of AV with the sensory test indicates that the shelf life of mayonnaise will be rejected when the AV is more than 10 g oleic acid kg fat$^{-1}$ week 1. The initial AV of both samples is 3.8. Predict the shelf lives of mayonnaise formulas 1 and 3 stored at 30 °C.

Solution: From the data in Table, the kinetic reaction can be described by a zero-order reaction. The kinetic rate constants (k) are applied in the Arrhenius model. The Arrhenius plot is presented in Figure. Table shows estimated kinetic parameters for the development of lipid oxidation during storage of different mayonnaise formulas. Figure shows the appearance of mayonnaise stored at 5, 35, and 55 °C. This sample was analyzed for rancidity retardation. However, the temperature at 55 C was not suitable for the shelf life study because the mayonnaise sample was rejected due to emulsion separation.

Table: Rate constants for lipid oxidation assuming zero-order reaction kinetics of different mayonnaise formulas.

| Formula | Propolis (%) | Fish oil (%) | k (g oleic acid kg fat$^{-1}$ week$^{-1}$) | | |
|---|---|---|---|---|---|
| | | | 5 °C | 35 °C | 55 °C |
| 1 | 0.00 | 0 | 0.153 | 0.396 | 0.494 |
| 2 | 0.25 | 0 | 0.188 | 0.369 | 0.489 |
| 3 | 0.50 | 0 | 0.098 | 0.237 | 0.343 |
| 4 | 0.00 | 2 | 0.308 | 0.410 | 0.410 |
| 5 | 0.25 | 2 | 0.288 | 0.356 | 0.437 |
| 6 | 0.50 | 2 | 0.368 | 0.439 | 0.576 |

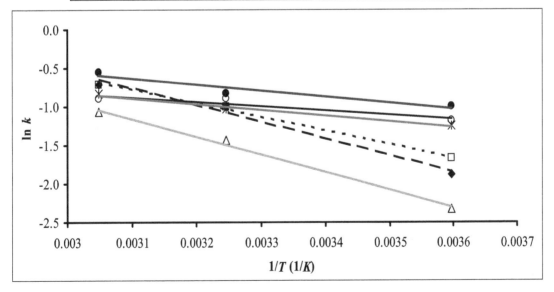

Arrhenius plot (ln k vs. 1/T ) for lipid oxidation (AV value) rate constants of different mayonnaise formulas during storage. A, 0% propolis and 0% fish oil; ,, 0.25% propolis and 0% fish oil; D, 0.5% propolis and 0% fish oil; B, 0% propolis and 2% fish oil; *, 0.25% propolis and 2% fish oil; C, 0.5% propolis and 2% fish oil.

Table: Estimated kinetic parameters for the development of lipid oxidation during storage of different mayonnaise formulas.

| Formula | Propolis (%) | Fish oil (%) | Ea (kJ mol$^{-1}$) | ln $k_0$ (g oleic acid kg fat$^{-1}$ week$^{-1}$) | $R^2$ |
|---|---|---|---|---|---|
| 1 | 0.00 | 0 | 18.1 | 5.99 | 0.98 |
| 2 | 0.25 | 0 | 14.7 | 4.69 | 0.99 |
| 3 | 0.50 | 0 | 19.2 | 6.01 | 0.99 |
| 4 | 0.00 | 2 | 4.6 | 0.85 | 0.87 |
| 5 | 0.25 | 2 | 6.2 | 1.41 | 0.98 |
| 6 | 0.50 | 2 | 6.5 | 1.78 | 0.92 |

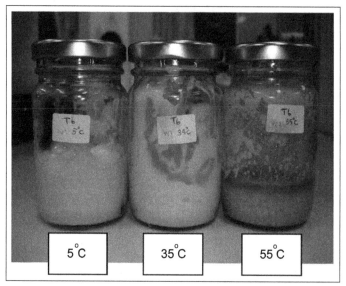

Mayonnaise appearance after storage at different temperatures.

Table: Shelf life prediction of mayonnaise formulas 1 and 3 stored at 30°C.

| Formula | ln k = ln $k_0$ - $E_a$/RT | k (g oleic acid kg fat$^{-1}$ week$^{-1}$) | A - $A_0$ =-kt | Shelf life (week) |
|---|---|---|---|---|
| 1 | -1.194 | -0.302 | (3.8-10)=(-0.302)*t | 20.5 |
| 2 | 1.611 | -0.199 | (3.8-10)=(-0.199)*t | 31.1 |

Results from this example showed that fish oil increased the development of lipid oxidation as reflected by a significantly (p < 0.05) higher AV. Addition of propolis extract significantly reduced (p < 0.05) the high AV. The predicted shelf lives of mayonnaise formulas 1 and 3 stored at 30 °C will be 20 and 31 weeks, respectively, as calculated in Table. This confirmed that the addition of 2% propolis can extend the shelf life of mayonnaise by ~11 weeks when compared to the control (no propolis).

# References

- Food-safety-and-the-different-types-of-food-contamination: foodsafety.com.au, Retrieved 09 March, 2019
- Investigation-and-identification-of-physical-contaminants-in-food: foodsafetymagazine.com, Retrieved 25 July, 2019
- Cross-contamination-prevention-995635: thespruceeats.com, Retrieved 29 June, 2019

- Shelf-Life-of-Foods- 28011534: academia.edu, Retrieved 14 February, 2019

- Techniques-in-Shelf-Life-Evaluation-of-Food-Products- 305385492: researchgate.net, Retrieved 26 January, 2019

- Valdes Biles P.; Ziobro G. C. (August 2000). "Regulatory Action Criteria for Filth and Other Extraneous Materials IV. Visual Detection of Hair in Food". Regulatory Toxicology and Pharmacology. Academic Press. 32 (1): 73–77. doi:10.1006/rtph.2000.1403. ISSN 0273-2300. PMID 11029271

- Garcha, S (September 2018). "Control of food spoilage molds using lactobacillus bacteriocins". Journal of Pure and Applied Microbiology. 12 (3): 1365–1373. doi:10.22207/JPAM.12.3.39

# 6

# Food Preservation

Food preservation is defined as the prevention of the growth of microorganisms and maintain food quality. It includes some methods such as fermentation, pasteurization, salting, pickling, canning, salting, etc. This chapter closely examines these methods of food preservation to provide an extensive understanding of the subject.

The term food preservation refers to any one of a number of techniques used to prevent food from spoiling. It includes methods such as canning, pickling, drying and freeze-drying, irradiation, pasteurization, smoking, and the addition of chemical additives. Food preservation has become an increasingly important component of the food industry as fewer people eat foods produced on their own lands, and as consumers expect to be able to purchase and consume foods that are out of season.

The vast majority of instances of food spoilage can be attributed to one of two major causes: (1) the attack by pathogens (disease-causing microorganisms) such as bacteria and molds, or (2) oxidation that causes the destruction of essential biochemical compounds and/or the destruction of plant and animal cells. The various methods that have been devised for preserving foods are all designed to reduce or eliminate one or the other (or both) of these causative agents.

For example, a simple and common method of preserving food is by heating it to some minimum temperature. This process prevents or retards spoilage because high temperatures kill or inactivate most kinds of pathogens. The addition of compounds known as BHA and BHT to foods also prevents spoilage in another different way. These compounds are known to act as antioxidants, preventing chemical reactions that cause the oxidation of food those results in its spoilage. Almost all techniques of preservation are designed to extend the life of food by acting in one of these two ways.

The search for methods of food preservation probably can be traced to the dawn of human civilization. People who lived through harsh winters found it necessary to find some means of insuring a food supply during seasons when no fresh fruits and vegetables were available. Evidence for the use of dehydration (drying) as a method of food preservation, for example, goes back at least 5,000 years. Among the most primitive forms of food preservation that are still in use today are such methods as smoking, drying, salting, freezing, and fermenting.

Early humans probably discovered by accident that certain foods exposed to smoke seem to last longer than those that are not. Meats, fish, fowl, and cheese were among such foods. It appears that compounds present in wood smoke have anti-microbial actions that prevent the growth of organisms that cause spoilage. Today, the process of smoking has become a sophisticated method of food preservation with both hot and cold forms in use. Hot smoking is used primarily with fresh or frozen foods, while cold smoking is used most often with salted products. The most advantageous conditions for each kind of smoking—air velocity, relative humidity, length of exposure, and salt content, for example—are now generally understood and applied during the smoking process. For example, electrostatic precipitators can be employed to attract smoke particles and improve the penetration of the particles into meat or fish. So many alternative forms of preservation are now available that smoking no longer holds the position of importance it once did with ancient peoples. More frequently, the process is used to add interesting and distinctive flavors to foods.

Because most disease-causing organisms require a moist environment in which to survive and multiply, drying is a natural technique for preventing spoilage. Indeed, the act of simply leaving foods out in the sun and wind to dry out is probably one of the earliest forms of food preservation. Evidence for the drying of meats, fish, fruits, and vegetables go back to the earliest recorded human history. At some point, humans also learned that the drying process could be hastened and improved by various mechanical techniques. For example, the Arabs learned early on that apricots could be preserved almost indefinitely by macerating them, boiling them, and then leaving them to dry on broad sheets. The product of this technique, quamar-adeen, is still made by the same process in modern Muslim countries.

Today, a host of dehydrating techniques are known and used. The specific technique adopted depends on the properties of the food being preserved. For example, a traditional method for preserving rice is to allow it to dry naturally in the fields or on drying racks in barns for about two weeks. After this period of time, the native rice is threshed and then dried again by allowing it to sit on straw mats in the sun for about three days. Modern drying techniques make use of fans and heaters in controlled environments. Such methods avoid the uncertainties that arise from leaving crops in the field to dry under natural conditions. Controlled temperature air drying is especially popular for the preservation of grains such as maize, barley, and bulgur.

Vacuum drying is a form of preservation in which a food is placed in a large container from which air is removed. Water vapor pressure within the food is greater than that outside of it, and water evaporates more quickly from the food than in a normal atmosphere. Vacuum drying is biologically desirable since some enzymes that cause oxidation of foods become active during normal air drying. These enzymes do not appear to be as active under vacuum drying conditions, however. Two of the special advantages of vacuum drying are that the process is more efficient at removing water from a food product, and it takes place more quickly than air drying. In one study, for example, the drying time of a fish fillet was reduced from about 16 hours by air drying to six hours as a result of vacuum drying.

Coffee drinkers are familiar with the process of dehydration known as spray drying. In this process, a concentrated solution of coffee in water is sprayed though a disk with many small holes in it. The surface area of the original coffee grounds is increased many times, making dehydration of the dry product much more efficient. Freeze-drying is a method of preservation that makes use of the physical principle known as sublimation. Sublimation is the process by which a solid passes directly to the gaseous phase without first melting. Freeze-drying is a desirable way of preserving food because at low temperatures (commonly around 14 °F to −13 °F [−10 °C to −25 °C]) chemical reactions take place very slowly and pathogens have difficulty surviving. The food to be preserved by this method is first frozen and then placed into a vacuum chamber. Water in the food first freezes and then sublimes, leaving a moisture content in the final product of as low as 0.5%.

The precise mechanism by which salting preserves food is not entirely understood. It is known that salt binds with water molecules and thus acts as a dehydrating agent in foods. A high level of salinity may also impair the conditions under which pathogens can survive. In any case, the value of adding salt to foods for preservation has been well known for centuries. Sugar appears to have effects similar to those of salt in preventing spoilage of food. The use of either compound (and of certain other natural materials) is known as curing. A desirable side effect of using salt or sugar as a food preservative is, of course, the pleasant flavor each compound adds to the final product.

Curing can be accomplished in a variety of ways. Meats can be submerged in a salt solution known as brine, for example, or the salt can be rubbed on the meat by hand. The injection of salt solutions into meats has also become popular. Food scientists have now learned that a number of factors relating to the food product and to the preservative conditions affect the efficiency of curing. Some of the food factors include the type of food being preserved, the fat content, and the size of treated pieces. Preservative factors include brine temperature and concentration, and the presence of impurities.

Curing is used with certain fruits and vegetables, such as cabbage (in the making of sauerkraut), cucumbers (in the making of pickles), and olives. It is probably most popular, however, in the preservation of meats and fish. Honey-cured hams, bacon, and corned beef ("corn" is a term for a form of salt crystals) are common examples.

Freezing is an effective form of food preservation because the pathogens that cause food spoilage are killed or do not grow very rapidly at reduced temperatures. The process is less effective in food preservation than are thermal techniques such as boiling because pathogens are more likely to be able to survive cold temperatures than hot temperatures. In fact, one of the problems surrounding the use of freezing as a method of food preservation is the danger that pathogens deactivated (but not killed) by the process will once again become active when the frozen food thaws.

A number of factors are involved in the selection of the best approach to the freezing of foods, including the temperature to be used, the rate at which freezing is to take place, and the actual method used to freeze the food. Because of differences in cellular composition, foods actually begin to freeze at different temperatures ranging from about 31 °F (−0.6 °C) for some kinds of fish to 19 °F (−7 °C) for some kinds of fruits.

The rate at which food is frozen is also a factor, primarily because of aesthetic reasons. The more slowly food is frozen, the larger the ice crystals that are formed. Large ice crystals have the tendency to cause rupture of cells and the destruction of texture in meats, fish, vegetables, and fruits. In order to deal with this problem, the technique of quick-freezing has been developed. In quick-freezing, a food is cooled to or below its freezing point as quickly as possible. The product thus obtained, when thawed, tends to have a firm, more natural texture than is the case with most slow-frozen foods.

About a half dozen methods for the freezing of foods have been developed. One, described as the plate, or contact, freezing technique, was invented by the American inventor Charles Birdseye in 1929. In this method, food to be frozen is placed on a refrigerated plate and cooled to a temperature less than its freezing point. Alternatively, the food may be placed between two parallel refrigerated plates and frozen. Another technique for freezing foods is by immersion in very cold liquids. At one time, sodium chloride brine solutions were widely used for this purpose. A 10% brine solution, for example, has a freezing point of about 21 °F (−6 °C), well within the desired freezing range for many foods. More recently, liquid nitrogen has been used for immersion freezing. The temperature of liquid nitrogen is about −320 °F (−195.5 °C), so that foods immersed in this substance freeze very quickly.

As with most methods of food preservation, freezing works better with some foods than with others. Fish, meat, poultry, and citrus fruit juices (such as frozen orange juice concentrate) are among the foods most commonly preserved by this method.

Fermentation is a naturally occurring chemical reaction by which a natural food is converted into another form by pathogens. It is a process in which food spoils, but results in the formation of an edible product. Perhaps the best example of such a food is cheese. Fresh milk does not remain in edible condition for a very long period of time. Its pH is such that harmful pathogens begin to grow in it very rapidly. Early humans discovered, however, that the spoilage of milk can be controlled in such a way as to produce a new product, cheese.

Bread is another food product made by the process of fermentation. Flour, water, sugar, milk, and other raw materials are mixed together with yeasts and then baked. The addition of yeasts brings about the fermentation of sugars present in the mixture, resulting in the formation of a product that will remain edible much longer than will the original raw materials used in the bread-making process.

Heating food is an effective way of preserving it because the great majority of harmful pathogens are killed at temperatures close to the boiling point of water. In this respect, heating foods is a form of food preservation comparable to that of freezing but much superior to it in its effectiveness. A preliminary step in many other forms of food preservation, especially forms that make use of packaging, is to heat the foods to temperatures sufficiently high to destroy pathogens.

In many cases, foods are actually cooked prior to their being packaged and stored. In other cases, cooking is neither appropriate nor necessary. The most familiar example of the latter situation is pasteurization. During the 1860s, the French bacteriologist Louis Pasteur discovered that pathogens in foods could be destroyed by heating those foods to a certain minimum temperature. The process was particularly appealing for the preservation of milk since preserving milk by boiling is not a practical approach. Conventional methods of pasteurization called for the heating of milk to a temperature between 145 and 149 °F (63-65 °C) for a period of about 30 minutes, and then cooling it to room temperature. In a more recent revision of that process, milk can also be "flash-pasteurized" by raising its temperature to about 160 °F (71 °C) for a minimum of 15 seconds, with equally successful results. A process known as ultra-high-pasteurization uses even higher temperatures, of the order of 194-266 °F (90-130 °C), for periods of a second or more.

One of the most common methods for preserving foods today is to enclose them in a sterile container. The term "canning" refers to this method although the specific container can be glass, plastic, or some other material as well as a metal can, from which the procedure originally obtained its name. The basic principle behind canning is that a food is sterilized, usually by heating, and then placed within an airtight container. In the absence of air, no new pathogens can gain access to the sterilized food. In most canning operations, the food to be packaged is first prepared—cleaned, peeled, sliced, chopped, or treated in some other way—and then placed directly into the container.

The container is then placed in hot water or some other environment where its temperature is raised above the boiling point of water for some period of time. This heating process achieves two goals at once. First, it kills the vast majority of pathogens that may be present in the container. Second, it forces out most of the air above the food in the container.

After heating has been completed, the top of the container is sealed. In home canning procedures, one way of sealing the (usually glass) container is to place a layer of melted paraffin directly on top of the food. As the paraffin cools, it forms a tight solid seal on top of the food. Instead of or in addition to the paraffin seal, the container is also sealed with a metal screw top containing a rubber gasket. The first glass jar designed for this type of home canning operation, the Mason jar, was patented in 1858.

The commercial packaging of foods frequently makes use of tin, aluminum, or other kinds of metallic cans. The technology for this kind of canning was first developed in the mid-1800s, when individual workers hand-sealed cans after foods had been cooked within them. At this stage, a single worker could seldom produce more than 100 "canisters" of food a day. With the development of far more efficient canning machines in the late nineteenth century, the mass production of canned foods became a reality.

As with home canning, the process of preserving foods in metal cans is simple in concept. The foods are prepared and the empty cans are sterilized. The prepared foods are then added to the sterile metal can, the filled can is heated to a sterilizing temperature, and the cans are then sealed by a machine. Modern machines are capable of moving a minimum of 1,000 cans per minute through the sealing operation.

The majority of food preservation operations used today also employ some kind of chemical additive to reduce spoilage. Of the many dozens of chemical additives available, all are designed either to kill or retard the growth of pathogens or to prevent or retard chemical reactions that result in the oxidation of foods. Some familiar examples of the former class of food additives are sodium benzoate and benzoic acid; calcium, sodium propionate, and propionic acid; calcium, potassium, sodium sorbate, and sorbic acid; and sodium and potassium sulfite. Examples of the latter class of additives include calcium, sodium ascorbate, and ascorbic acid (vitamin C); butylated hydroxyanisole (BHA) and buty-lated hydroxytoluene (BHT); lecithin; and sodium and potassium sulfite and sulfur dioxide.

A special class of additives that reduce oxidation is known as the sequestrants. Sequestrants are compounds that "capture" metallic ions, such as those of copper, iron, and nickel, and remove them from contact with foods. The removal of these ions helps preserve foods because in their free state they increase the rate at which oxidation of foods takes place. Some examples of sequestrants used as food preservatives are ethylenediamine-tetraacetic acid (EDTA), citric acid, sorbitol, and tartaric acid.

# Food Preservatives

All food products except for the one growing in your kitchen garden have food preservatives in them. Every manufacturer adds food preservative to the food during processing. The purpose is generally to avoid spoilage during the transportation time.

Food is so important for the survival, so food preservation is one of the oldest technologies used by human beings to avoid its spoilage. Different ways and means have been found and improved for the purpose. Boiling, freezing & refrigeration, pasteurizing, dehydrating, pickling are the traditional few. Sugar, mineral salt and salt are also often used as preservatives food. Nuclear radiation is also being used now as food preservatives. Modified packaging techniques like vacuum packing and hypobaric packing also work as food preservatives.

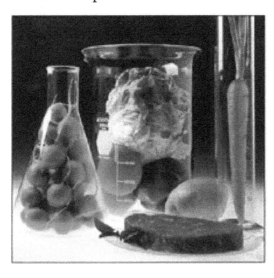

Food preservation is basically done for three reasons:

- To preserve the natural characteristics of food.

- To preserve the appearance of food.

- To increase the shelf value of food for storage.

## Natural Food Preservatives

In the category of natural food preservatives comes the salt, sugar, alcohol, vinegar etc. These are the traditional preservatives in food that are also used at home while making pickles, jams and juices etc. Also the freezing, boiling, smoking, salting are considered to be the natural ways of preserving food. Coffee powder and soup are dehydrated and freeze-dried for preservation. The citrus food preservatives like citrus acid and ascorbic acid work on enzymes and disrupt their metabolism leading to the preservation.

Sugar and salt are the earliest natural food preservatives that very efficiently drops the growth of bacteria in food. To preserve meat and fish, salt is still used as a natural food preservative.

## Chemical Food Preservatives

Chemical food preservatives are also being used for quite some time now. They seem to be the best and the most effective for a longer shelf life and are generally fool proof for the preservation purpose. Examples of chemical food preservatives are:

- Benzoates (such as sodium benzoate, benzoic acid),

- Nitrites (such as sodium nitrite),

- Sulphites (such as sulphur dioxide),

- Sorbates (such as sodium sorbate, potassium sorbate.

Antioxidants are also the chemical food preservatives that act as free radical scavengers. In this category of preservatives in food comes the vitamin C, BHA (butylated hydroxyanisole), bacterial growth inhibitors like sodium nitrite, sulfur dioxide and benzoic acid.

Then there is ethanol that is a one of the chemical preservatives in food, wine and food stored in brandy. Unlike natural food preservatives some of the chemical food preservatives are harmful. Sulfur dioxide and nitrites are the examples. Sulfur dioxide causes irritation in bronchial tubes and nitrites are carcinogenic.

## Artificial Preservatives

Artificial preservatives are the chemical substances that stop of delayed the growth of bacteria, spoilage and its discoloration. These artificial preservatives can be added to the food or sprayed on the food.

## Types of Artificial Preservatives in Food

- Antimicrobial agents,

- Antioxidants,

- Chelating agents.

In antimicrobial comes the Benzoates, Sodium benzoate, Sorbates and Nitrites. Antioxidants include the Sulfites, Vitamin E, Vitamin C and Butylated hydroxytoluene (BHT) Chelating agent has the Disodium ethylenediaminetetraacetic acid (EDTA), Polyphosphates and Citric acid.

## Harmful Food Preservatives

Although preservatives food additives are used to keep the food fresh and to stop the bacterial growth. But still there are certain preservatives in food that are harmful if taken in more than the prescribed limits.

- Benzoates: This group of chemical food preservative has been banned in Russia because of its role in triggering allergies, asthma and skin rashes. It is also considered to cause the brain damage. This food preservative is used in fruit juices, tea, coffee etc.

- Butylates: This chemical food preservative is expected to cause high blood pressure and cholestrol level. This can affect the kidney and live function. It is found in butter, vegetable oils and margarine.

- BHA (butylated hydroxyanisole): BHA is expected to cause the live diseases and cancer. This food preservative is used to preserve the fresh pork and pork sausages, potato chips, instant teas, cake mixes and many more.

- Caramel: Caramel is the coloring agent that causes the vitamin B6 deficiencies, genetic effects and cancer. It is found in candies, bread, brown colored food and frozen pizza.

In addition to this there are many other harmful food preservatives. These are Bromates, Caffeine, Carrageenan, Chlorines, Coal Tar AZO Dies, Gallates, Glutamates, Mono- and Di-glycerides, Nitrates/Nitrites, Saccharin, Sodium Erythrobate, Sulphites and Tannin.

## Preservatives as Food Additives

All of these chemicals act as either antimicrobials or antioxidants or both. They either inhibit the activity of or kill the bacteria, molds, insects and other microorganisms. Antimicrobials prevent the growth of molds, yeasts and bacteria and antioxidants keep foods from becoming rancid or developing black spots. They suppress the reaction when foods come in contact with oxygen, heat, and some metals. They also prevent the loss of some essential amino acids some vitamins.

Table: Some common preservatives and their primary activity.

| Chemical Affected | Organism(s) | Action | Use in Foods |
|---|---|---|---|
| Sulfites | Insects & Microorganisms | Antioxidant | Dried Fruits, Wine, Juice |
| Sodium Nitrite | Clostridia | Antimicrobial | Cured Meats |
| Propionic Acid | Molds | Antimicrobial | Bread, Cakes, Cheeses |
| Sorbic Acid | Molds | Antimicrobial | Cheeses, Cakes, Salad Dressing |
| Benzoic Acid | Yeasts & Molds | Antimicrobial | Soft Drinks, Ketchup, Salad Dressings |

There are other antioxidants like Sodium Erythorbate, Erythorbic Acid, Sodium Diacetate, Sodium Succinate, Grape Seed Extract, Pine Bark Extract, Apple Extract Tea Proplyphenols, Succinic Acid and Ascorbic Acid and food preservatives like Parabens and Sodium Dehydro Acetate used frequently for preservation.

## Frozen Food

Freezing food preserves it from the time it is prepared to the time it is eaten. Since early times, farmers, fishermen, and trappers have preserved grains and produce in unheated buildings during the winter season. Freezing food slows down decomposition by turning residual moisture into ice, inhibiting the growth of most bacterial species. In the food commodity industry, there are two processes: mechanical and cryogenic (or flash freezing). The freezing kinetics is important to preserve the food quality and texture. Quicker freezing generates smaller ice crystals and maintains cellular structure. Cryogenic freezing is the quickest freezing technology available due to the ultra low liquid nitrogen temperature –196 °C (–320 °F).

Preserving food in domestic kitchens during modern times is achieved using household freezers. Accepted advice to householders was to freeze food on the day of purchase. An initiative by a supermarket group in 2012 (backed by the UK's Waste & Resources Action Programme) promotes the freezing of food "as soon as possible up to the product's 'use by' date". The Food Standards Agency was reported as supporting the change, provided the food had been stored correctly up to that time.

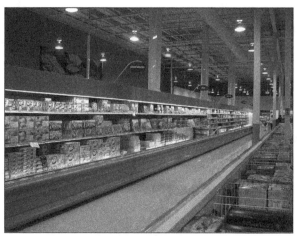

A frozen processed foods aisle at a supermarket.

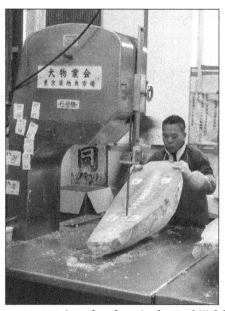

Cutting frozen tuna using a bandsaw in the Tsukiji fish market.

## Preservatives

Frozen products do not require any added preservatives because microorganisms do not grow when the temperature of the food is below −9.5 °C (15 °F), which is sufficient on its own in preventing food spoilage. Long-term preservation of food may call for food storage at even lower temperatures. Carboxymethylcellulose (CMC), a tasteless and odorless stabilizer, is typically added to frozen food because it does not adulterate the quality of the product.

## Technology

The freezing technique itself, just like the frozen food market, is developing to become faster, more efficient and more cost-effective.

Mechanical freezers were the first to be used in the food industry and are used in the vast majority of freezing / refrigerating lines. They function by circulating a refrigerant, normally ammonia, around the system, which withdraws heat from the food product. This heat is then transferred to a condenser and dissipated into air or water. The refrigerant itself, now a high pressure, hot liquid, is directed into an evaporator. As it passes through an expansion valve, it is cooled and then vaporises into a gaseous state. Now a low pressure, low temperature gas again, it can be reintroduced into the system.

Cryogenic (or flash freezing) of food is a more recent development, but is used by many leading food manufacturers all over the world. Cryogenic equipment uses very low temperature gases – usually liquid nitrogen or solid carbon dioxide – which are applied directly to the food product.

## Packaging

Frozen food packaging must maintain its integrity throughout filling, sealing, freezing, storage, transportation, thawing, and often cooking. As many frozen foods are cooked in a microwave oven, manufacturers have developed packaging that can go straight from freezer to the microwave.

In 1974, the first differential heating container (DHC) was sold to the public. A DHC is a sleeve of metal designed to allow frozen foods to receive the correct amount of heat. Various sized apertures were positioned around the sleeve. The consumer would put the frozen dinner into the sleeve according to what needed the most heat. This ensured proper cooking.

Today there are multiple options for packaging frozen foods. Boxes, cartons, bags, pouches, Boil-in-Bags, lidded trays and pans, crystallized PET trays, and composite and plastic cans.

Scientists are continually researching new aspects of frozen food packaging. Active packaging offers a host of new technologies that can actively sense and then neutralize the presence of bacteria or other harmful species. Active packaging can extend shelf-life, maintain product safety, and help preserve the food over a longer period of time. Several functions of active packaging are being researched:

- Oxygen scavengers,

- Time temperature indicators and digital temperature data loggers,

- Antimicrobials,

- Carbon dioxide controllers,

- Microwave susceptors,

- Moisture control: Water activity, Moisture vapor transmission rate,

- Flavor enhancers,

- Odor generators,

- Oxygen-permeable films,

- Oxygen generators.

## Effects on Nutrients

### Vitamin Content of Frozen Foods

- Vitamin C: Usually lost in a higher concentration than any other vitamin. A study was performed on peas to determine the cause of vitamin C loss. A vitamin loss of ten percent occurred during the blanching phase with the rest of the loss occurring during the cooling and washing stages. The vitamin loss was not actually accredited to the freezing process. Another experiment was performed involving peas and lima beans. Frozen and canned vegetables were both used in the experiment. The frozen vegetables were stored at −23 °C (−10 °F) and the canned vegetables were stored at room temperature 24 °C (75 °F). After 0, 3, 6, and 12 months of storage, the vegetables were analyzed with and without cooking. O'Hara, the scientist performing the experiment said, "From the view point of the vitamin content of the two vegetables when they were ready for the plate of the consumer, there did not appear to be any marked advantages attributable to method of preservation, frozen storage, processed in a tin, or processed in glass."

- Vitamin $B_1$ (Thiamin): A vitamin loss of 25 percent is normal. Thiamin is easily soluble in water and is destroyed by heat.

- Vitamin $B_2$ (Riboflavin): Not much research has been done to see how much freezing affects Riboflavin levels. Studies that have been performed are inconclusive; one study found an 18 percent vitamin loss in green vegetables, while another determined a 4 percent loss. It is commonly accepted that the loss of Riboflavin has to do with the preparation for freezing rather than the actual freezing process itself.

- Vitamin A (Carotene): There is little loss of carotene during preparation for freezing and freezing of most vegetables. Much of the vitamin loss is incurred during the extended storage period.

### Effectiveness

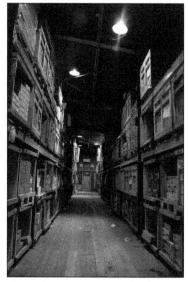

A frozen food warehouse at McMurdo Station, Antarctica.

Freezing is an effective form of food preservation because the pathogens that cause food spoilage are killed or do not grow very rapidly at reduced temperatures. The process is less effective in food preservation than are thermal techniques, such as boiling, because pathogens are more likely to be able to survive cold temperatures rather than hot temperatures. One of the problems surrounding the use of freezing as a method of food preservation is the danger that pathogens deactivated (but not killed) by the process will once again become active when the frozen food thaws.

Foods may be preserved for several months by freezing. Long-term frozen storage requires a constant temperature of −18 °C (0 °F) or less.

## Defrosting

To be used, many cooked foods that have been previously frozen require defrosting prior to consumption. Preferably, some frozen meats should be defrosted prior to cooking to achieve the best outcome: cooked through evenly and of good texture.

Ideally, most frozen foods should be defrosted in a refrigerator to avoid significant growth of pathogens. However, this can take considerable time.

Food is often defrosted in one of several ways:

- At room temperature; this is dangerous since the outside may be defrosted while the inside remains frozen.

- In a refrigerator.

- In a microwave oven.

- Wrapped in plastic and placed in cold water or under cold running water.

People sometimes defrost frozen foods at room temperature because of time constraints or ignorance; such foods should be promptly consumed after cooking or discarded and never be refrozen or refrigerated since pathogens are not killed by the freezing process.

## Quality

The speed of the freezing has a direct impact on the size and the number of ice crystals formed within a food product's cells and extracellular space. Slow freezing leads to fewer but larger ice crystals while fast freezing leads to smaller but more numerous ice crystals. Large ice crystals can puncture the walls of the cells of the food product which will cause a degradation of the texture of the product as well as the loss of its natural juices during thawing. That is why there will be a qualitative difference observed between food products frozen by ventilated mechanical freezing, non-ventilated mechanical freezing or cryogenic freezing with liquid nitrogen.

# Fermentation

Fermentation in food processing is the process of converting carbohydrates to alcohol or organic acids using microorganisms—yeasts or bacteria—under anaerobic conditions. Fermentation usually implies that the action of microorganisms is desired. The science of fermentation is known as zymology or zymurgy.

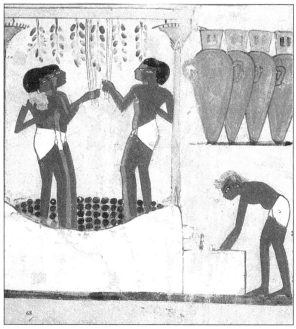

Grapes being trodden to extract the juice and made into wine in storage jars.

The term fermentation sometimes refers specifically to the chemical conversion of sugars into ethanol, producing alcoholic drinks such as wine, beer, and cider. However, similar processes take place in the leavening of bread ($CO_2$ produced by yeast activity), and in the preservation of sour foods with the production of lactic acid, such as in sauerkraut and yogurt.

Other widely consumed fermented foods include vinegar, olives, and cheese. More localised foods prepared by fermentation may also be based on beans, grain, vegetables, fruit, honey, dairy products, fish.

## Uses

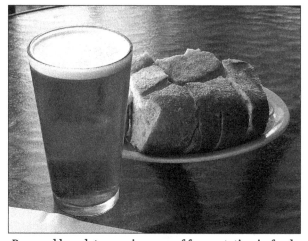

Beer and bread, two major uses of fermentation in food.

Food fermentation is the conversion of sugars and other carbohydrates into alcohol or preservative organic acids and carbon dioxide. All three products have found human uses. The production of alcohol is made use of when fruit juices are converted to wine, when grains are made into beer, and when foods rich in starch, such as potatoes, are fermented and then distilled to make spirits such as gin and vodka. The production of carbon dioxide is used to leaven bread. The production of organic acids is exploited to preserve and flavor vegetables and dairy products.

Food fermentation serves five main purposes: to enrich the diet through development of a diversity of flavors, aromas, and textures in food substrates; to preserve substantial amounts of food through lactic acid, alcohol, acetic acid, and alkaline fermentations; to enrich food substrates with protein, essential amino acids, and vitamins; to eliminate antinutrients; and to reduce cooking time and the associated use of fuel.

## Risks

Alaska has witnessed a steady increase of cases of botulism since 1985. It has more cases of botulism than any other state in the United States of America. This is caused by the traditional Eskimo practice of allowing animal products such as whole fish, fish heads, walrus, sea lion, and whale flippers, beaver tails, seal oil, and birds, to ferment for an extended period of time before being consumed. The risk is exacerbated when a plastic container is used for this purpose instead of the old-fashioned, traditional method, a grass-lined hole, as the *Clostridium botulinum* bacteria thrive in the anaerobic conditions created by the air-tight enclosure in plastic.

The World Health Organization has classified pickled foods as possibly carcinogenic, based on epidemiological studies. Other research found that fermented food contains a carcinogenic by-product, ethyl carbamate (urethane). "A 2009 review of the existing studies conducted across Asia concluded that regularly eating pickled vegetables roughly doubles a person's risk for esophageal squamous cell carcinoma."

## High Pressure Treatment in Foods

Currently consumers worldwide are more demanding with regard to the quality and safety of the foods they consume, especially those that produce the perception of healthy products. To meet these demands, the food industry has improved its heat preservation processes by developing continuous high temperature/short time (HTST) and ultra-high temperature (UHT) treatments and aseptic packaging. In addition, consumption of minimally processed products has increased significantly. These products maintain a high standard of nutrition and flavor, while meeting the required safety level and achieving a long shelf life.

Minimally processed foods have been developed alongside the development of various emerging preservation technologies. Within this group of technologies there are the so-called "non-thermal preservation technologies," which do not use heat as the main form of microbial and enzyme inactivation. Although heat is generated by some of these processes, the temperature increase never reaches the levels of a conventional thermal process and can be suitably controlled by a cooling station. These new preservation technologies include oscillatory magnetic fields, pulsed electric fields, ultrasound, irradiation, and high hydrostatic pressure. Probably the most developed and most widely implanted technology at the industrial level is high hydrostatic pressure. This technology has demonstrated its capability of preserving sensory and nutritional qualities of foods while producing suitable levels of microbiological and enzyme inactivation.

## High Hydrostatic Pressure Technology

The main objective of any non-thermal technology is to maximize the freshness and flavor qualities of the foodstuffs while achieving the required level of food safety. High hydrostatic pressure (HHP) meets with these requirements and today it being incorporated in many companies as an alternative to conventional heat treatment procedures. Applications include the preservation of meat products, oysters, fruit jams, fruit juices, salad dressings, fresh calamari, rice cake, duck liver, jam, guacamole, and many ready-to-eat foods. In all these cases, microbial and enzyme inactivation is achieved without altering the product quality. In relation to the total percentage utilization of HHP equipment, vegetable products account for 28%, meat products for 26%, sea foods and fish for 15%, juices and beverages for 14%, and other products for 17%, generating an amount of 350,000,000 kg of processed products in 2012, according to data from Hiperbaric, S.A.

All this makes HHP the most commercially developed non-thermal technology, with very good acceptance by consumers, who value the organoleptic characteristics of pressure-treated products with a quality barely affected by treatment. Currently the world market has experienced significant growth in the incorporation of equipment at industrial level.

In general, microbial inactivation is achieved at pressures that vary from 100 to 800 MPa during relatively short times (from a few seconds to several minutes). Some treatments are combined with mild temperatures between 20 and 50 °C to inactivate enzymes. The processing conditions depend fundamentally on the food to be treated and the microorganisms and enzymes to be inactivated; we note that this technology at the pressure currently used in the food industry does not inactivate bacterial spores.

## Packaging

The package is an important part in the development and industrial application of HHP as a preservation technology. It is possible to use a great variety of packages with different shapes; however, food must be packed in a flexible and resistant package, able to withstand pressure and maintain the integrity. Polyethylene (PE), polyethylene terephthalate (PET), polypropylene (PP), ethylene-vinyl alcohol (EVOH), polyamide (PA), and nylon films are some of the packaging materials currently used in industrial food processing by HHP treatments. Juliano et al. suggest minimize the headspace up to 30% to maximize the utilization of the vessel capacity and minimize the time needed for preheating, if the treatment requires temperature. Usually, an HPP vessel will utilize its 50%–70% volume capacity depending on the shape of the package and the vessel design.

## Microbial Inactivation

The objective of any preservation process is the inactivation of microorganisms that can spoil the food and/or produce illness in the consumer (pathogenic microorganisms). The response of microorganisms to HHP has been extensively studied varies according to the following factors: Molds and yeasts are the most sensitive microorganisms; Gram-negative bacteria have medium sensitivity, whereas Gram-positive bacteria are the most resistant among vegetative cells and their spores need very high pressures to be inactivated. Regarding the action mechanisms of pressure, according to the studies carried out by Huang et al. a pressure of 50 MPa can affect or inhibit protein synthesis and produce a reduction in the number of microbial ribosomes. A pressure of 100 MPa can cause partial denaturalization of cellular proteins; when the pressure is increased to 200 MPa it produces internal damage in the microbial structure and external damage in the cellular membrane. Pressures equal or similar to 300 MPa produce irreversible damage to the microorganism, including leakage of intracellular components to the surrounding medium, resulting finally in cellular death.

The various effects that take place in microorganisms depend on their physiological state, microorganisms in log phase being more sensitive to HHP than those in stationary phase. This behavior could be explained by the fact that in the log phase the microorganism is in the process of cellular division and the membrane is more sensitive to environmental stresses. This effect was also reported by Mañas and Mackay in Escherichia coli strain J1, in exponential and stationary phases. The cells in stationary phase showed higher resistance to HHP treatment than those in exponential phase. Some modifications were also observed (aggregation of cytoplasmic proteins, condensation of the nucleoid) after 200 MPa treatments for 8 min at 20 °C.

Temperature is a very important environmental stress in HHP treatments because the combination of the two technologies, with short times can increases significantly microbial inactivation. According to studies carried out by Chen and Hoover and Ross et al., an HHP treatment of *L. monocytogenes* at initial temperatures of 45–50 °C and 5 min produced more than 5 log decimal reductions in the initial microbial concentration in UHT whole milk. However, was necessary to increase the treatment time to 35 min to produce the same inactivation at initial temperature of 22 °C.

HHP has proved to be an effective technology for inactivating various pathogens, as reported by Jofré et al. The application of a treatment of 600 MPa for 6 min at 31 °C resulted in a reduction close to 3.5 decimal log for E. coli, Listeria monocytogenes, Salmonella enterica subsp. enterica, Yersinia enterocolitica, and Campylobacter jejuni in meat products.

Although there are many studies in relation to the effect of HHP on bacteria, the information that exists on molds and yeasts is relatively scarce. In general, yeasts and molds can be inactivated at 200–400 MPa, but when they are in the spore or ascospore state or in a food with a very high concentration of sugar the pressure needed to inactivate them could be close to 600 MPa. These microorganisms are frequently involved in spoilage of cereals derivatives (tofu, tortillas), minimally processed vegetables, and lactic derivatives such as butter, yoghurt, and soft cheese.

Table: High hydrostatic pressure (HHP) inactivation of molds and yeasts in different foods.

| Food product | Microorganism | HHP conditions | Inactivation results |
|---|---|---|---|
| Pineapple juice | Byssochlamys nivea | 550–600 MPa for 3–15 min at 20–80 °C. | 600 MPa for 15 min at 80 °C, 5.7 log reduction. |
| Apple-broccoli juice | S. cerevisiae; A. flavus | 250–400 MPa for 5–20 min at 21 °C. | 400 MPa for 10 min at 21 °C, 5 log reduction. |

| Apple juice | Talaromyces avellaneus | 200–600 MPa for 10–60 min at 17–60 °C. | 600 MPa for 50 min at 60 °C, 5 log reduction ascospores. |
| Concentrated orange juice | S. cerevisiae | 100–400 MPa for 0–120 min at 20 °C. | 400 MPa for 60 min at 20 °C, 3 log reduction. |
| Cheese | P. roqueforti | 50–800 MPa for 20 min at 10–30 °C. | 400 MPa for 20 min at 20 °C, 6 log reduction. |

## Spore Inactivation

Spores are cellular forms that some microorganisms have developed as a response to adverse environmental situations in order to survive. Spores are characterized by their high resistance to different environmental stresses and preservation treatments. The most important spore-producing genera are Clostridium, Bacillus and Alicyclobacillus. The initial spore load present in foods can be significantly reduced by HHP in combination with mild temperatures. In various published studies, 3.5 decimal log reductions have been reported for Clostridium sporogenes and 5.7 decimal log reductions for Bacillus coagulans by HHP at temperatures of 60–90 °C. Furthermore, Meyer observed significant reductions in the initial spore concentration in low-acid foods after treatments ranging between 700 and 1000 MPa and a product temperature of 70 °C. With those conditions they obtained foods that were microbiologically stable at room temperature, and in many cases the quality of the products was higher than that of those processed by heat.

Table: HHP inactivation of spores in different foods.

| Food product | Microorganism | HHP conditions | Inactivation results |
|---|---|---|---|
| Carrot juice | B. licheniformis | 400–600 MPa for 0–40 min at 40–60 °C. | 241 to 465 MPa (D value range 23.3 to 31 °C). |
| Cooked chicken | C. botulinum | 600 MPa for 2 min at 20 °C. | 600 MPa for 2 min at 20 °C, 2 log reduction. |
| Orange juice | A. acidoterrestris | 200–600 MPa for 1–15 min at 45–65 °C. | 600 MPa, D55 °C = 7 min; 200 MPa, D65 °C = 5.0 min. |
| Tomato sauce | B. coagulans; A. acidoterrestris | 100–800 MPa for 10 min at 25, 40, 60 °C. | 700 MPa for 10 min at 60 °C, 2 log reduction. |
| Tomato pulp | B. coagulans | 300–600 MPa for 0–39 min at 50–60 °C. | 600 MPa for 15 at 60 °C 5.7 log reduction. |
| Orange Juice | A. acidoterrestris | 200–600 MPa for 10 min at 20–60 °C. | 600 MPa for 10 min at 50 °C, 3 log reduction. |
| Milk | B. sporothermodurans | 300–500 MPa for 10–30 min at 30–50 °C. | 495 MPa for 30 min at 49 °C, 5 log reduction. |

At present, methods to germinate spores before HHP treatment are under study. Exist different methods for germination of spores such as combining extremely high pressure and temperature, methods that involves using low or medium pressure (150–300 MPa), temperature, and other factors as single amino acids, sugars, asparagine, glucose, fructose to germinate the spores and produce bacterial vegetative cells, after which the bacterial vegetative cells are inactivate using HHP. In addition, there are other germinant agents, which include lysozyme, salts, and cationic surfactants such as dodecylamine that can be used in combination with high pressure. It is important to point out however that the spores of proteolytic Clostridium botulinum and Clostridium sporogenes germinate in response to l-alanine but not to universal germinant AGFK (a mixture of l-asparagine, d-glucose, d-fructose, and potassium ions) or inosine. This initial process can be followed by HHP treatment of 300–900 MPa at 30–60 °C.

According to the study carried out by Georget et al. to germinate Geobacillus stearothermophilusspores under moderate high pressure in buffer N-(2-acetamido)-2-aminoethanesulfonic acid (ACES) applying a treatment of 200 MPa with temperature of 55 °C , an inactivation over 2 log10 was achieved after 5 min of treatment. A 200 MPa for 40 min at 55 °C treatment led an inactivation of 3 log reduction following the subsequent inactivation to 80 °C for 20 min. In case of the spores of Clostridium botulinumearlier studies in cooked chicken with 2% sodium lactate, showed that germination of spores occurred at 4 °C and a spore reduction in the initial inoculum of 1.7 log10 cfu/g with a treatment at 600 MPa for 2 min at 20 °C was achieved. For the germination and inactivation of Clostridium perfringens spores in poultry meat, spores were incubated for 15 min at 55 °C with an addition of l-asparagine and potassium chloride, followed of a treatment of 568 MPa at 73 °C for 10 min achieving ~4 log reductions in the concentration of spores.

## Effects of HHP on Proteins

HHP technology has been used fundamentally to reduce the microbial load and increase the safety and shelf life of treated foods with superior nutritional and sensory properties to those thermally treated. Nevertheless, the effect of HHP on proteins has raised interest and studies have been carried out to elucidate it. High Hydrostatic Pressure treatments affect the non-covalent links (ionic, hydrophobic, and hydrogen links) of proteins, which means that the secondary, tertiary, and quaternary structures can be unfolded and dissociated while the primary structure remains stable. Messens et al. reported that it is necessary to apply a pressure of around 150 MPa to observe changes in the quaternary structure, and it is necessary to apply more than 200 MPa to significantly modify the secondary and tertiary structures. Owing to these changes, Liu et al. and Tabilo-Munizaga et al. studied the application of this technology to develop industrial applications to confer unique characteristics to foods (gel formation, emulsions, foams, new flavors and textures) or to seek a fat replacement. The possibility of using these new products as fat replacements has encouraged in-depth studies of stabilizing and gelling agents, agents that are usually incorporated in foodstuffs to give stability, texture, and palatability. It is important to note that the changes depend directly on the type of protein used (disulfide bridges, linked by hydrophobic interactions, isoelectric points) and the HHP treatment (pressure, time, and temperature). All these studies make HHP a promising technology for the revalorization of waste and agro-industrial by-products.

According to He et al., when proteins isolated from peanuts were treated at pressures between 50 and 200 MPa for 5 min the isolates increased their water-holding capacity (WHC) and oil-binding capacity (OBC), producing changes of interest in relation to protein properties. Additionally, the effect of HHP on milk proteins and whey has been studied in depth under various treatment conditions. The results indicated various changes in protein structure. Casein micelles experienced significant changes at pressures between 150 and 400 MPa and at a temperature of 20 °C. However, a greater denaturalization of proteins from whey β-lactoglobulin and α-lactalbumin was observed at pressures higher than 100 and 400 MPa, respectively.

The effect of pressure on vegetable proteins has also been studied. Protein isolates from peanuts (5% w/v of protein) produced gels at 100 MPa for 5 min at 25 °C, while isolates from soya protein (9% w/v of protein) produced gels at 600 MPa for 5 to 10 min and a temperature of 33.5 °C. For gelification of the isolates it was necessary to add $CaCl_2$ at a concentration of 0.015–0.020 mol $L^{-1}$, in accordance with the work reported by Maltais et al., who indicated that calcium concentrations are very important and determine the final characteristics of gels. At low calcium concentrations filamentous gels occurred, while at high concentrations disordered phase separation gels or aggregates appeared.

## Effect of HHP on Enzymes

There are two important regions in an enzyme, one responsible for recognizing the substrate and the other responsible for catalyzing the reaction when joined to the substrate. Minimal conformational change in the structure may completely affect the enzyme functionality.

Enzymes can be divided into two groups according to the effect of treatment by high hydrostatic pressure. In the first group are enzymes that are activated with pressures of 100–500 MPa, an activation that occurs only in monomeric proteins. The second group includes enzymes that are inactivated when exposed to pressures higher than 500 MPa in combination with relatively high temperatures. The main studies conducted on the effect of HHP on enzymes are based on the enzymes that are most often present in foodstuffs and produce deterioration of it or unacceptable sensory changes. Among them we can highlight the enzymes peroxidase (POD), pectin methylesterase (PME), lipoxygenase (LOX), and polyphenol oxidase (PPO), as shown in the study carried out by Ludikhuyze et al. In general, polyphenol oxidase (PPO) and peroxidase (POD) are inactivated by applying a pressure equal to or greater than 400 MPa in combination with temperatures between 20 and 90 °C. Under these conditions, enzyme activity can be reduced by up to 50%, although the percentages may vary depending on the intrinsic properties of processed foods. It should be noted that the predictive models used in thermal inactivation are often inadequate to describe inactivation by HHP treatment.

Table: HHP inactivation of enzymes in different foods.

| Food product | Enzyme | HHP conditions | Inactivation achieved |
|---|---|---|---|
| Jam | Pectin methylesterase (PME); Peroxidase (POD) | 550–700 MPa for 2.5–75 min at 45–75 °C | PME: 27%–40% POD: 51%–70% |
| Feijoa puree | Peroxidase (POD); Polyphenol oxidase (PPO); Pectin methylesterase (PME) | 600 MPa for 5 min at 25 °C | POD: 78% PPO: 55.6% PME: 56% |
| Camarosa strawberry | Polyphenol oxidase (PPO) | 600 MPa for 15 min at 34–62 °C | PPO: 82% |
| Fruit smoothies | Polyphenol oxidase (PPO) | 600 MPa for 10 min at 20 °C | PPO: 83% |
| Dry-cured ham | Glutathione peroxidase (GSHPx); Superoxide dismutase (SOD) | 900 MPa for 5 min at 12 °C | GSHPx: 44.2% SOD: 17.6% |
| Strawberry pulps | β-Glucosidase; Polyphenol oxidase (PPO); Peroxidase (POD) | 400–600 MPa for 5–25 min at 25 °C | β-Glu: 41.4% PPO: 74.6% POD: 74.6% |

## Some Industrial Applications of HHP

HHP technology has become a commercially implemented technology in fruit juice processing, spreading from its origins in Japan to the USA and Europe, and now Australia, with worldwide utilization increasing almost exponentially since 2000. In the U.S., Genesis Juice Corp.® processes eight types of organic juices by HHP, including apple, carrot, apple-ginger, apple-strawberry, ginger lemonade, strawberry lemonade, a herbal tea beverage, and apple- and banana-based smoothies, other company of high interest by its increment in sales in U.S., is Suja™, situated in San Diego, CA, produces a variety of mixture vegetable and fruits juices. European companies presently employing this technology in fruit juice processing include Invo® making smoothies in Spain, UltiFruit® making orange and grapefruit juices and a mixture of strawberry-orange juice in France, Frubaça® manufacturing various fruit-based beverages in Portugal, Juicy Line-Fruity Line® in Holland, Beskyd Frycovice, a.s® manufacturing mixtures of broccoli-apple-lemon and broccoli-orange-lemon in the Czech Republic, ATA S.P.A.® manufacturing carrot and apple juices in Italy, and Puro® commercializing smoothies in the UK.

Regarding processing conditions, treatments are optimized at a pressure level of 600 MPa in combination with moderate heat. In addition, due to the special characteristics of fruit juices, (nutritional components, flavor) and the perception by the consumer as a healthy food, quantities ranging from 500 to 2000 kg/h can be produced to satisfy current consumer demand considering the current capacities of industrial equipment. Shelf lives are estimated at ca. 10–35 day under refrigeration conditions, depending on the type of juice. Products are sold in supermarket chains, specialty and gourmet stores, and food services providing fruit preparations and dressings. Two main packaging formats are used, a small volume containing 250 mL, corresponding to a single portion, and a larger format containing 1 L.

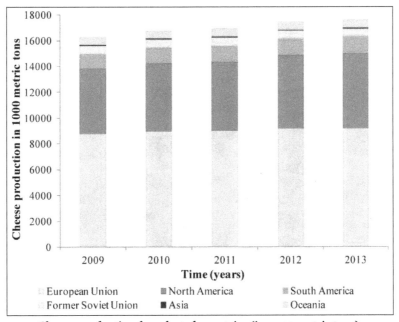

Cheese production for selected countries (in 1000 metric tons).

One application of HHP that has great appeal is the stabilization of fresh cheese due its global consumption and the increase in global production of 3.5 million tons in the last 10 years, the cheese belongs to the ready-to-eat (RTE) food group, this product is characterized by special physical and chemical properties such as a near neutral pH, high water activity of 0.97, and high relative humidity, and is very prone to contamination from pathogens such as Staphylococcus aureus, Listeria monocytogenes, Salmonella spp., Escherichia coli O157:H7, and spoilage microorganisms, such as molds and yeasts. Although currently this type of fresh cheese is made from pasteurized milk, the microbial recontamination occurs during subsequent processes, commonly in the stages of handling and packaging. That is why high hydrostatic pressure technology could be of great interest in the microbiological stabilization of this product, avoiding high annual losses from foodborne diseases in which fresh cheeses are involved and rejections due to spoilage.

# Food Irradiation

Food irradiation is the process of exposing food and food packaging to ionizing radiation. Ionizing radiation, such as from gamma rays, x-rays, or electron beams, is energy that can be transmitted without direct contact to the source of the energy (radiation) capable of freeing electrons from their atomic bonds (ionization) in the targeted food. The radiation can be emitted by a radioactive substance or generated electrically. This treatment is used to improve food safety by extending product shelf-life (preservation), reducing the risk of foodborne illness, delaying or eliminating sprouting or ripening, by sterilization of foods, and as a means of controlling insects and invasive pests. Food irradiation primarily extends the shelf-life of irradiated foods by effectively destroying organisms responsible for spoilage and foodborne illness and inhibiting sprouting.

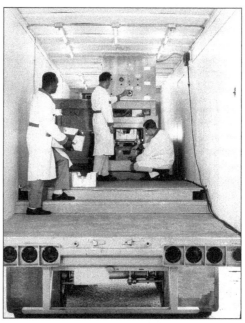

A portable, trailer-mounted food irradiation machine.

Although consumer perception of foods treated with irradiation is more negative than those processed by other means, because people imagine that the food is radioactive or mutated, these thoughts don't agree with the understood mechanism by which irradiation works. The food itself is already not alive, so irradiation will not affect it meaningfully. Irradiation will kill the living bacteria, however. Additionally, all independent research, the U.S. Food and Drug Administration (FDA), the World Health Organization (WHO), the Centers for Disease Control and Prevention (CDC), and U.S. Department of Agriculture (USDA) have performed studies that confirm irradiation to be safe. In order for a food to be irradiated in the US, the FDA will still require that the specific food be thoroughly tested for irradiation safety.

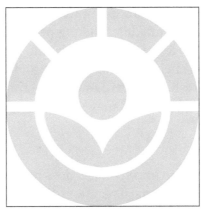

The international Radura logo, used to show a food has been treated with ionizing radiation.

Food irradiation is permitted by over 60 countries, with about 500,000 metric tons of food annually processed worldwide. The regulations that dictate how food is to be irradiated, as well as the food allowed to be irradiated, vary greatly from country to country. In Austria, Germany, and many other countries of the European Union only dried herbs, spices, and seasonings can be processed with irradiation and only at a specific dose, while in Brazil all foods are allowed at any dose.

## Uses

Irradiation is used to reduce or eliminate the risk of food-borne illnesses, prevent or slow down spoilage, arrest maturation or sprouting and as a treatment against pests. Depending on the dose, some or all of the pathogenic organisms, microorganisms, bacteria, and viruses present are destroyed, slowed down, or rendered incapable of reproduction. Irradiation cannot return spoiled or over-ripe food to a fresh state. If this food was processed by irradiation, further spoilage would cease and ripening would slow down, yet the irradiation would not destroy the toxins or repair the texture, color, or taste of the food. When targeting bacteria, most foods are irradiated to significantly reduce the number of active microbes, not to sterilize all microbes in the product. In this respect it is similar to pasteurization.

Irradiation is used to create safe foods for people at high risk of infection, or for conditions where food must be stored for long periods of time and proper storage conditions are not available. Foods that can tolerate irradiation at sufficient doses are treated to ensure that the product is completely sterilized. This is most commonly done with rations for astronauts, and special diets for hospital patients.

Irradiation is used to create shelf-stable products. Since irradiation reduces the populations of spoilage microorganisms, and because pre-packed food can be irradiated, the packaging prevents recontamination of the final product.

Irradiation is used to reduce post-harvest losses. It reduces populations of spoilage micro-organisms in the food and can slow down the speed at which enzymes change the food, and therefore slows spoilage and ripening, and inhibits sprouting (e.g., of potato, onion, and garlic).

Food is also irradiated to prevent the spread of invasive pest species through trade in fresh vegetables and fruits, either within countries, or trade across international boundaries. Pests such as insects could be transported to new habitats through trade in fresh produce which could significantly affect agricultural production and the environment were they to establish themselves. This "phytosanitary irradiation" aims to render any hitch-hiking pest incapable of breeding. The pests are sterilized when the food is treated by low doses of irradiation. In general, the higher doses required to destroy pests such as insects, mealybugs, mites, moths, and butterflies either affect the look or taste, or cannot be tolerated by fresh produce. Low dosage treatments (less than 1000 gray) enables trade across quarantine boundaries and may also help reduce spoilage.

## Impact

Irradiation reduces the risk of infection and spoilage, does not make food radioactive, and the food is shown to be safe, but it does cause chemical reactions that alter the food and therefore alters the chemical makeup, nutritional content, and the sensory qualities of the food. Some of the potential secondary impacts of irradiation are hypothetical, while others are demonstrated. These effects include cumulative impacts to pathogens, people, and the environment due to the reduction of food quality, the transportation and storage of radioactive goods, and destruction of pathogens, changes in the way we relate to food and how irradiation changes the food production and shipping industries.

## Immediate Effects

The radiation source supplies energetic particles or waves. As these waves/particles pass through a target material they collide with other particles. Around the sites of these collisions chemical bonds are broken, creating short lived radicals (e.g. the hydroxyl radical, the hydrogen atom and solvated electrons). These radicals cause further chemical changes by bonding with and or stripping particles from nearby molecules. When collisions damage DNA or RNA, effective reproduction becomes unlikely, also when collisions occur in cells, cell division is often suppressed.

Irradiation (within the accepted energy limits, as 10 MeV for electrons, 5 MeV for X-rays [US 7.5 MeV] and gamma rays from Cobalt-60) can not make food radioactive, but it does produce radiolytic products, and free radicals in the food. A few of these products are unique, but not considered dangerous.

Irradiation can also alter the nutritional content and flavor of foods, much like cooking. The scale of these chemical changes is not unique. Cooking, smoking, salting, and other less novel techniques, cause the food to be altered so drastically that its original nature is almost unrecognizable, and must be called by a different name. Storage of food also causes dramatic chemical changes, ones that eventually lead to deterioration and spoilage.

## Misconceptions

A major concern is that irradiation might cause chemical changes that are harmful to the consumer. Several national expert groups and two international expert groups evaluated the available data and concluded that any food at any dose is wholesome and safe to consume as long as it remains palatable and maintains its technical properties (e.g. feel, texture, or color).

Irradiated food does not become radioactive, just as an object exposed to light does not start producing light. Radioactivity is the ability of a substance to emit high energy particles. When particles hit the target materials they may free other highly energetic particles. This ends shortly after the end of the exposure, much like objects stop reflecting light when the source is turned off and warm objects emit heat until they cool down but do not continue to produce their own heat. To modify a material so that it keeps emitting radiation (induce radiation) the atomic cores (nucleus) of the atoms in the target material must be modified.

It is impossible for food irradiators to induce radiation in a product. Irradiators emit electrons or photons and the radiation is intrinsically radiated at precisely known strengths (wavelengths for photons, and speeds for electrons). These radiated particles at these strengths can never be strong enough to modify the nucleus of the targeted atom in the food, regardless of how many particles hit the target material, and radioactivity can not be induced without modifying the nucleus.

## Chemical Changes

Compounds known as free radicals form when food is irradiated. Most of these are oxidizers (i.e., accept electrons) and some react very strongly. According to the free-radical theory of aging excessive amounts of these free radicals can lead to cell injury and cell death, which may contribute to many diseases. However, this generally relates to the free radicals generated in the body, not the free radicals consumed by the individual, as much of these are destroyed in the digestive process.

Most of the substances found in irradiated food are also found in food that has been subjected to other food processing treatments, and are therefore not unique. One family of chemicals (2ACB's) are uniquely formed by irradiation (unique radiolytic products), and this product is nontoxic. When fatty acids are irradiated, a family of compounds called 2-alkylcyclobutanones (2-ACBs) are produced. These are thought to be unique radiolytic products. When irradiating food, all other chemicals occur in a lower or comparable frequency to other food processing techniques. Furthermore, the quantities in which they occur in irradiated food are lower or similar to the quantities formed in heat treatments.

The radiation doses to cause toxic changes are much higher than the doses used during irradiation, and taking into account the presence of 2-ACBs along with what is known of free radicals, these results lead to the conclusion that there is no significant risk from radiolytic products.

## Food Quality

Ionizing radiation can change food quality but in general very high levels of radiation treatment (many thousands of gray) are necessary to adversely change nutritional content, as well as the sensory qualities (taste, appearance, and texture). Irradiation to the doses used commercially to treat food have very little negative impact on the sensory qualities and nutrient content in foods. When irradiation is used to maintain food quality for a longer period of time (improve the shelf stability of some sensory qualities and nutrients) the improvement means that more consumers have access to the original taste, texture, appearance, and nutrients. The changes in quality and nutrition depend on the degree of treatment and may vary greatly from food to food.

There has been low level gamma irradiation that has been attempted on arugula, spinach, cauliflower, ash gourd, bamboo shoots, coriander, parsley, and watercress. There has been limited information, however, regarding the physical, chemical and/or bioactive properties and the shelf life on these minimally processed vegetables.

There is some degradation of vitamins caused by irradiation, but is similar to or even less than the loss caused by other processes that achieve the same result. Other processes like chilling, freezing, drying, and heating also result in some vitamin loss.

The changes in the flavor of fatty foods like meats, nuts and oils are sometimes noticeable, while the changes in lean products like fruits and vegetables are less so. Some studies by the irradiation industry show that for some properly treated fruits and vegetables irradiation is seen by consumers to improve the sensory qualities of the product compared to untreated fruits and vegetables.

## Quality Impact on Minimally Processed Vegetables

Watercress (*Nasturtium Officinale*) is a rapidly growing aquatic or semi aquatic perennial plant. Because chemical agents do not provide efficient microbial reductions, watercress has been tested with gamma irradiation treatment in order to improve both safety and the shelf life of the product. It is traditionally used on horticultural products to prevent sprouting and post-packaging contamination, delay post-harvest ripening, maturation and senescence.

In a Food Chemistry food journal, scientists studied the suitability of gamma irradiation of 1, 2, and 5 kGy for preserving quality parameters of the fresh cut watercress at around 4 degrees Celsius for 7 days. They determined that a 2 kGy dose of irradiation was the dose that contained most similar qualities to non-stored control samples, which is one of the goals of irradiation. 2 kGy preserved high levels of reducing sugars and favoured polyunsaturated fatty acids (PUFA); while samples of the 5 kGy dose revealed high contents of sucrose and monounsaturated fat (MUFA). Both cases the watercress samples obtained healthier fatty acids profiles. However, a 5kGy dose better preserved the antioxidant activity and total flavonoids.

## Long-term Impacts

If the majority of food was irradiated at high-enough levels to significantly decrease its nutritional content, there would be an increased risk of developing nutritionally-based illnesses if additional steps, such as changes in eating habits, were not taken to mitigate this. Furthermore, for at least three studies on cats, the consumption of irradiated food was associated with a loss of tissue in the myelin sheath, leading to reversible paralysis. Researchers suspect that reduced levels of vitamin A and high levels of free radicals may be the cause. This effect is thought to be specific to cats and has not been reproduced in any other animal. To produce these effects, the cats were fed solely on food that was irradiated at a dose at least five times higher than the maximum allowable dose.

It may seem reasonable to assume that irradiating food might lead to radiation-tolerant strains, similar to the way that strains of bacteria have developed resistance to antibiotics. Bacteria develop a resistance to antibiotics after an individual uses antibiotics repeatedly. Much like pasteurization plants, products that pass through irradiation plants are processed once, and are not processed and reprocessed. Cycles of heat treatment have been shown to produce heat-tolerant bacteria, yet no problems have appeared so far in pasteurization plants. Furthermore, when the irradiation dose is chosen to target a specific species of microbe, it is calibrated to doses several times the value required to target the species. This ensures that the process randomly destroys all members of a target species. Therefore, the more irradiation-tolerant members of the target species are not given any evolutionary advantage. Without evolutionary advantage, selection does not occur. As to the irradiation process directly producing mutations that lead to more virulent, radiation-resistant strains, the European Commission's Scientific Committee on Food found that there is no evidence; on the contrary, irradiation has been found to cause loss of virulence and infectivity, as mutants are usually less competitive and less adapted.

## Misconceptions

Some who advocate against food irradiation argue the safety of irradiated food is not scientifically proven because there are a lack of long-term studies in spite of the fact that hundreds of animal feeding studies of irradiated food, including multigenerational studies, have been performed since 1950. Endpoints investigated have included subchronic and chronic changes in metabolism, histopathology, function of most systems, reproductive effects, growth, teratogenicity, and mutagenicity. A large number of studies have been performed; meta-studies have supported the safety of irradiated food.

The below experiments are cited by food irradiation opponents, but either could not be verified in later experiments, could not be clearly attributed to the radiation effect, or could be attributed to an inappropriate design of the experiment.

India's National Institute of Nutrition (NIN) found an elevated rate of cells with more than one set of genes (polyploidy) in humans and animals when fed wheat that was irradiated recently (within 12 weeks). Upon analysis, scientists determined that the techniques used by the NIN allowed for too much human error and statistical variation; therefore, the results were unreliable. After multiple studies by independent agencies and scientists, no correlation between polyploidy and irradiation of food could be found.

## Indirect Effects of Irradiation

The indirect effects of irradiation are the concerns and benefits of irradiation that are related to how making food irradiation a common process will change the world, with emphasis on the system of food production.

If irradiation were to become common in the food handling process there would be a reduction of the prevalence of foodborne illness and potentially the eradication of specific pathogens. However, multiple studies suggest that an increased rate of pathogen growth may occur when irradiated food is cross-contaminated with a pathogen, as the competing spoilage organisms are no longer present. This being said, cross contamination itself becomes less prevalent with an increase in usage of irradiated foods.

The ability to remove bacterial contamination through post-processing by irradiation may reduce the fear of mishandling food which could cultivate a cavalier attitude toward hygiene and result in contaminants other than bacteria. However, concerns that the pasteurization of milk would lead to increased contamination of milk were prevalent when mandatory pasteurization was introduced, but these fears never materialized after adoption of this law. Therefore, it is unlikely for irradiation to cause an increase of illness due to nonbacteria-based contamination.

## Treatment

Up to the point where the food is processed by irradiation, the food is processed in the same way as all other food. To treat the food, they are exposed to a radioactive source, for a set period of time to achieve a desired dose. Radiation may be emitted by a radioactive substance, or by X-ray and electron beam accelerators. Special precautions are taken to ensure the food stuffs never come in contact with the radioactive substances and that the personnel and the environment are protected from exposure radiation. Irradiation treatments are typically classified by dose (high, medium, and low), but are sometimes classified by the effects of the treatment (radappertization, radicidation and radurization). Food irradiation is sometimes referred to as "cold pasteurization" or "electronic pasteurization" because ionizing the food does not heat the food to high temperatures during the process, and the effect is similar to heat pasteurization. The term "cold pasteurization" is controversial because the term may be used to disguise the fact the food has been irradiated and pasteurization and irradiation are fundamentally different processes.

Treatment costs vary as a function of dose and facility usage. A pallet or tote is typically exposed for several minutes to hours depending on dose. Low-dose applications such as disinfestation of fruit range between US$0.01/lbs and US$0.08/lbs while higher-dose applications can cost as much as US$0.20/lbs.

## Packaging

Food processors and manufacturers today struggle with using affordable, efficient packaging materials for irradiation based processing. The implementation of irradiation on prepackaged foods has been found to impact foods by inducing specific chemical alterations to the food packaging material that migrates into the food. Cross-linking in various plastics can lead to physical and chemical modifications that can increase the overall molecular weight. On the other hand, chain scission is fragmentation of polymer chains that leads to a molecular weight reduction.

## Dosimetry

The radiation absorbed dose is the amount energy absorbed per unit weight of the target material. Dose is used because, when the same substance is given the same dose, similar changes are observed in the target material. The SI unit for dose is grays (Gy or J/kg). Dosimeters are used to measure dose, and are small components that, when exposed to ionizing radiation, change measurable physical attributes to a degree that can be correlated to the dose received. Measuring dose (dosimetry) involves exposing one or more dosimeters along with the target material.

For purposes of legislation doses are divided into low (up to 1 kGy), medium (1 kGy to 10 kGy), and high-dose applications (above 10 kGy). High-dose applications are above those currently permitted in the US for commercial food items by the FDA and other regulators around the world. Though these doses are approved for non-commercial applications, such as sterilizing frozen meat for NASA astronauts (doses of 44 kGy) and food for hospital patients.

Table: Applications of food irradiation.

|  | Application | Dose (kGy) |
|---|---|---|
| Low dose (up to 1 kGy) | Inhibit sprouting (potatoes, onions, yams, garlic). | 0.06 - 0.2 |
|  | Delay in ripening (strawberries, potatoes). | 0.5 - 1.0 |
|  | Prevent insect infestation (grains, cereals, coffee beans, spices, dried nuts, dried fruits, dried fish, mangoes, papayas). | 0.15 -1.0 |
|  | Parasite control and inactivation (tape worm, trichina). | 0.3 - 1.0 |
| Medium dose (1 kGy to 10 kGy) | Extend shelf-life (raw and fresh fish, seafood, fresh produce, refrigerated and frozen meat products). | 1.0 - 7.0 |
|  | Reduce risk of pathogenic and spoilage microbes (meat, seafood, spices, and poultry). | 1.0 - 7.0 |
|  | Increased juice yield, reduction in cooking time of dried vegetables. | 3.0 - 7.0 |
| High dose (above 10 kGy) | Enzymes (dehydrated). | 10.0 |
|  | Sterilization of spices, dry vegetable seasonings. | 30.0 max |
|  | Sterilization of packaging material. | 10.0 - 25.0 |
|  | Sterilization of foods (NASA and hospitals). | 44.0 |

## Processes

## Gamma Irradiation

Gamma irradiation is produced from the radioisotopes cobalt-60 and caesium-137, which are derived by neutron bombardment of cobalt-59 and as a nuclear source by-product, respectively. Cobalt-60 is the most common source of gamma rays for food irradiation in commercial scale facilities as it is water insoluble and hence has little risk of environmental contamination by leakage into the water systems. As for transportation of the radiation source, cobalt-60 is transported in special trucks that prevent release of radiation and meet standards mentioned in the Regulations for Safe Transport of Radioactive Materials of the International Atomic Energy Act. The special trucks must meet high safety standards and pass extensive tests to be approved to ship radiation sources. Conversely, caesium-137, is water soluble and poses a risk of environmental contamination. Insufficient quantities are available for large scale commercial use. An incident where water-soluble caesium-137 leaked into the source storage pool requiring NRC intervention has led to near elimination of this radioisotope.

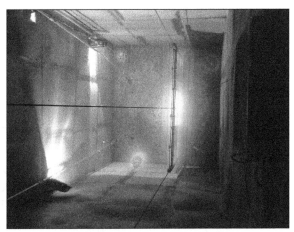

Cobalt 60 stored in Gamma Irradiation machine.

Gamma irradiation is widely used due to its high penetration depth and dose uniformity, allowing for large-scale applications with high through puts. Additionally, gamma irradiation is significantly less expensive than using an X-ray source In most designs, the radioisotope, contained in stainless steel pencils, is stored in a water-filled storage pool which absorbs the radiation energy when not in use. For treatment, the source is lifted out of the storage tank, and product contained in totes is passed around the pencils to achieve required processing.

## Electron Beam

Treatment of electron beams is created as a result of high energy electrons in an accelerator that generates electrons accelerated to 99% the speed of light. This system uses electrical energy and can be powered on and off. The high power correlates with a higher throughput and lower unit cost, but electron beams have low dose uniformity and a penetration depth of centimeters. Therefore, electron beam treatment works for products that have low thickness.

## X-ray

X-rays are produced by bombardment of dense target material with high energy accelerated electrons(this process is known as bremsstrahlung-conversion), giving rise to a continuous energy spectrum. Heavy metals, such as tantalum and tungsten, are used because of their high atomic numbers and high melting temperatures. Tantalum is usually preferred versus tungsten for industrial, large-area, high-power targets because it is more workable than tungsten and has a higher threshold energy for induced reactions. Like electron beams, x-rays do not require the use of radioactive materials and can be turned off when not in use. X-rays have high penetration depths and high dose uniformity but they are a very expensive source of irradiation as only 8% of the incident energy is converted into X-rays.

## Cost

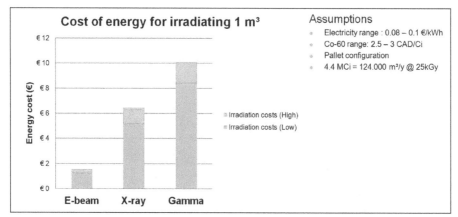

Efficiency illustration of the different radiation technologies (electron beam, X-ray, gamma rays).

The cost of food irradiation is influenced by dose requirements, the food's tolerance of radiation, handling conditions, i.e., packaging and stacking requirements, construction costs, financing arrangements, and other variables particular to the situation. Irradiation is a capital-intensive technology requiring a substantial initial investment, ranging from $1 million to $5 million. In the case of large research or contract irradiation facilities, major capital costs include a radiation source, hardware (irradiator, totes and conveyors, control systems, and other auxiliary equipment), land (1 to 1.5 acres), radiation shield, and warehouse. Operating costs include salaries (for fixed and variable labor), utilities, maintenance, taxes/insurance, cobalt-60 replenishment, general utilities, and miscellaneous operating costs. Perishable food items, like fruits, vegetables and meats would still require to be handled in the cold chain, so all other supply chain costs remain the same.

# Pasteurization

Pasteurization or pasteurisation is a process in which water and certain packaged and non-packaged foods (such as milk and fruit juice) are treated with mild heat, usually to less than 100 °C (212 °F), to eliminate pathogens and extend shelf life. The process is intended to destroy or deactivate organisms and enzymes that contribute to spoilage or risk of disease, including vegetative bacteria, but not bacterial spores. Since pasteurization is not sterilization, and does not kill spores, a second "double" pasteurization will extend the quality by killing spores that have germinated.

The process was named after the French scientist Louis Pasteur, whose research in the 1880s demonstrated that thermal processing would inactivate unwanted microorganisms in wine. Spoilage enzymes are also inactivated during pasteurization. Today, pasteurization is used widely in the dairy industry and other food processing industries to achieve food preservation and food safety.

Most liquid products are heat treated in a continuous system where heat can be applied using a plate heat exchanger and/or the direct or indirect use of hot water and steam. Due to the mild heat, there are minor changes to the nutritional quality and sensory characteristics of the treated foods. Pascalization or high pressure processing (HPP) and pulsed electric field (PEF) are non-thermal processes that are also used to pasteurize foods.

## Pasteurization Process

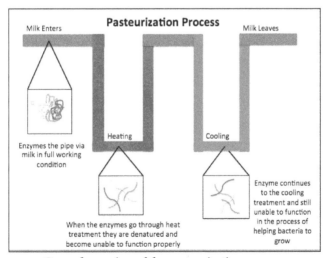

General overview of the pasteurization process.

The milk starts at the left and enters the piping with functioning enzymes that, when heat-treated, become denatured and stop the enzymes from functioning. This helps to stop pathogen growth by stopping the functionality of the cell. The cooling process helps stop the milk from undergoing the Maillard reaction and caramelization. The pasteurization process also has the ability to heat the cells to the point that they burst from pressure build-up.

Pasteurization is a mild heat treatment of liquid foods (both packaged and unpackaged) where products are typically heated to below 100 °C. The heat treatment and cooling process are designed to inhibit a phase change of the product. The acidity of the food determines the parameters (time and temperature) of the heat treatment as well as the duration of shelf life. Parameters also take into account nutritional and sensory qualities that are sensitive to heat.

In acidic foods (pH <4.6), such as fruit juice and beer, the heat treatments are designed to inactivate enzymes (pectin methylesterase and polygalacturonase in fruit juices) and destroy spoilage microbes (yeast and lactobacillus). Due to the low pH of acidic foods, pathogens are unable to grow. The shelf-life is thereby extended several weeks. In less acidic foods (pH >4.6), such as milk and liquid eggs, the heat treatments are designed to destroy pathogens and spoilage organisms (yeast and molds). Not all spoilage organisms are destroyed under pasteurization parameters, thus subsequent refrigeration is necessary.

## Equipment

Food can be pasteurized in two ways: either before or after being packaged into containers. When food is packaged in glass, hot water is used to lower the risk of thermal shock. Plastics and metals are also used to package foods, and these are generally pasteurized with steam or hot water since the risk of thermal shock is low.

Most liquid foods are pasteurized using continuous systems that have a heating zone, hold tube, and cooling zone, after which the product is filled into the package. Plate heat exchangers are used for low-viscosity products such as animal milks, nut milks and juices. A plate heat exchanger is composed of many thin vertical stainless steel plates which separate the liquid from the heating or cooling medium. Scraped surface heat exchangers contain an inner rotating shaft in the tube, and serve to scrape highly viscous material which might accumulate on the wall of the tube.

Shell or tube heat exchangers are designed for the pasteurization of Non-Newtonian foods such as dairy products, tomato ketchup and baby foods. A tube heat exchanger is made up of concentric stainless steel tubes. Food passes through the inner tube while the heating/cooling medium is circulated through the outer or inner tube.

The benefits of using a heat exchanger to pasteurize non-packaged foods versus pasteurizing foods in containers are:

- Heat exchangers provides uniform treatment, and there is greater flexibility with regards to the products which can be pasteurized on these plates.

- The process is more energy-efficient compared to pasteurizing foods in packaged containers.

- Greater throughput.

After being heated in a heat exchanger, the product flows through a hold tube for a set period of time to achieve the required treatment. If pasteurization temperature or time is not achieved, a flow diversion valve is utilized to divert under-processed product back to the raw product tank. If the product is adequately processed, it is cooled in a heat exchanger, then filled.

High-temperature short-time (HTST) pasteurization, such as that used for milk (71.5 °C (160.7 °F) for 15 seconds) ensures safety of milk and provides a refrigerated shelf life of approximately two weeks. In ultra-high-temperature (UHT) pasteurization, milk is pasteurized at 135 °C (275 °F) for 1–2 seconds, which provides the same level of safety, but along with the packaging, extends shelf life to three months under refrigeration.

## Verification

Direct microbiological techniques are the ultimate measurement of pathogen contamination, but these are costly and time-consuming, which means that products have a reduced shelf-life by the time pasteurization is verified.

As a result of the unsuitability of microbiological techniques, milk pasteurization efficacy is typically monitored by checking for the presence of alkaline phosphatase, which is denatured by pasteurization. Destruction of alkaline phosphatase ensures the destruction of common milk pathogens. Therefore, the presence of alkaline phosphatase is an ideal indicator of pasteurization efficacy. For liquid eggs, the effectiveness of the heat treatment is measured by the residual activity of α-amylase.

### Efficacy against Pathogenic Bacteria

During the early 20th century, there was no robust knowledge of what time and temperature combinations would inactivate pathogenic bacteria in milk, and so a number of different pasteurization standards were in use. By 1943, both HTST pasteurization conditions of 72 °C (162 °F) for 15 seconds, as well as batch pasteurization conditions of 63 °C (145 °F) for 30 minutes, were confirmed by studies of the complete thermal death (as best as could be measured at that time) for a range of pathogenic bacteria in milk. Complete inactivation of *Coxiella burnetii* (which was thought at the time to cause Q fever by oral ingestion of infected milk) as well as of *Mycobacterium tuberculosis* (which causes tuberculosis) were later demonstrated. For all practical purposes, these conditions were adequate for destroying almost all yeasts, molds, and common spoilage bacteria and also for ensuring adequate destruction of common pathogenic, heat-resistant organisms. However, the microbiological techniques used until the 1960s did not allow for the actual reduction of bacteria to be enumerated. Demonstration of the extent of inactivation of pathogenic bacteria by milk pasteurization came from a study of surviving bacteria in milk that was heat-treated after being deliberately spiked with high levels of the most heat-resistant strains of the most significant milk-borne pathogens.

The mean $\log_{10}$ reductions and temperatures of inactivation of the major milk-borne pathogens during a 15-second treatment are:

- *Staphylococcus aureus* > 6.7 at 66.5 °C (151.7 °F).

- *Yersinia enterocolitica* > 6.8 at 62.5 °C (144.5 °F).

- Pathogenic *Escherichia coli* > 6.8 at 65 °C (149 °F).

- *Cronobacter sakazakii* > 6.7 at 67.5 °C (153.5 °F).

- *Listeria monocytogenes* > 6.9 at 65.5 °C (149.9 °F).

- Salmonella ser. Typhimurium > 6.9 at 61.5 °C (142.7 °F).

The Codex Alimentarius *Code of Hygienic Practice for Milk* notes that milk pasteurization is designed to achieve at least a 5 $\log_{10}$ reduction of *Coxiella burnetii*. The Code also notes that: "The minimum pasteurization conditions are those having bactericidal effects equivalent to heating every particle of the milk to 72 °C for 15 seconds (continuous flow pasteurization) or 63 °C for 30 minutes (batch pasteurization)" and that "To ensure that each particle is sufficiently heated, the milk flow in heat exchangers should be turbulent, *i.e.* the Reynolds number should be sufficiently high." The point about turbulent flow is important because simplistic laboratory studies of heat inactivation that use test tubes, without flow, will have less bacterial inactivation than larger-scale experiments that seek to replicate conditions of commercial pasteurization.

As a precaution, modern HTST pasteurization processes must be designed with flow-rate restriction as well as divert valves which ensure that the milk is heated evenly and that no part of the milk is subject to a shorter time or a lower temperature. It is common for the temperatures to exceed 72 °C by 1.5 °C or 2 °C.

## Effects on Nutritional and Sensory Characteristics of Foods

Because of its mild heat treatment, pasteurization increases the shelf-life by a few days or weeks. However, this mild heat also means there are only minor changes to heat-labile vitamins in the foods.

## Milk

According to a systematic review and meta-analysis, it was found that pasteurization appeared to reduce concentrations of vitamins B12 and E, but it also increased concentrations of vitamin A. Apart from meta-analysis, it is not possible to draw conclusions about the effect of pasteurization on vitamins A, B12, and E based merely on consultation of the vast literature available. Milk is not an important source of vitamins B12 or E in the North American diet, so the effects of pasteurization on the adult daily intake of these vitamins is negligible. However, milk is considered an important source of vitamin A, and because pasteurization appears to increase vitamin A concentrations in milk, the effect of milk heat treatment on this vitamin is a not a major public health concern. Results of meta-analyses reveal that pasteurization of milk leads to a significant decrease in vitamin C and folate, but milk is also not an important source of these vitamins. A significant decrease in vitamin B2 concentrations was found after pasteurization. Vitamin B2 is typically found in bovine milk at concentrations of 1.83 mg/liter. Because the recommended daily intake for adults is 1.1 mg/day, milk consumption greatly contributes to the recommended daily intake of this vitamin. With the exception of B2, pasteurization does not appear to be a concern in diminishing the nutritive value of milk because milk is often not a primary source of these studied vitamins in the North American diet.

## Sensory Effects

Pasteurization also has a small but measurable effect on the sensory attributes of the foods that are processed. In fruit juices, pasteurization may result in loss of volatile aroma compounds. Fruit juice products undergo a deaeration process prior to pasteurization that may be responsible for this loss. Deaeration also minimizes the loss of nutrients like vitamin C and carotene. To prevent the decrease in quality resulting from the loss in volatile compounds, volatile recovery, though costly, can be utilized to produce higher-quality juice products.

In regards to color, the pasteurization process does not have much effect on pigments such as chlorophylls, anthocyanins and carotenoids in plants and animal tissues. In fruit juices, polyphenol oxidase (PPO) is the main enzyme responsible for causing browning and color changes. However, this enzyme is deactivated in the deaeration step prior to pasteurization with the removal of oxygen.

In milk, the color difference between pasteurized and raw milk is related to the homogenization step that takes place prior to pasteurization. Before pasteurization, milk is homogenized to separate the solids (fat) from the liquid, which results in the pasteurized milk having a whiter appearance compared to raw milk. For vegetable products, color degradation is dependent on the temperature conditions and the duration of heating.

Pasteurization may result in some textural loss as a result of enzymatic and non-enzymatic transformations in the structure of pectin if the processing temperatures are too high as a result. However, with mild heat treatment pasteurization, tissue softening in the vegetables that causes textural loss is not of concern as long as the temperature does not get above 80 °C (176 °F).

## Novel Pasteurization Methods

Other thermal and non-thermal processes have been developed to pasteurize foods as a way of reducing the effects on nutritional and sensory characteristics of foods and preventing degradation of heat-labile nutrients. Pascalization or high pressure processing (HPP) and pulsed electric field (PEF) are examples of these non-thermal pasteurization methods that are currently commercially utilized.

Microwave volumetric heating (MVH) is the newest available pasteurization technology. It uses microwaves to heat liquids, suspensions, or semi-solids in a continuous flow. Because MVH delivers energy evenly and deeply into the whole body of a flowing product, it allows for gentler and shorter heating, so that almost all heat-sensitive substances in the milk are preserved.

Low Temperature, Short Time (LTST) is a patented method that implies spraying droplets in a chamber heated below the usual pasteurization temperatures. It takes several thousandth of a second to treat liquid products, so the method is also known as the millisecond technology (MST). It significantly extends the shelf life of products (50+ days) when combined with HTST without damaging the nutrients or flavor. LTST has been commercial since 2019.

## Products that are Commonly Pasteurized

- Beer,
- Canned food,

- Dairy products,

- Eggs,

- Milk,

- Juices,

- Low alcoholic beverages,

- Syrups,

- Vinegar,

- Water,

- Wines,

- Nuts.

## Pickling

Pickling is the process of preserving or extending the lifespan of food by either anaerobic fermentation in brine or immersion in vinegar. In East Asia, vinaigrette (vegetable oil and vinegar) is also used as a pickling medium. The pickling procedure typically affects the food's texture, taste and flavor. The resulting food is called a *pickle*, or, to prevent ambiguity, prefaced with *pickled*. Foods that are pickled include vegetables, fruits, meats, fish, dairy and eggs.

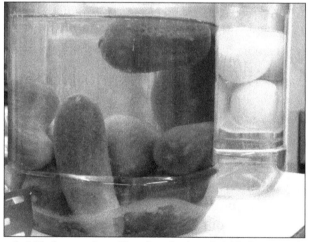

A jar of pickled cucumbers (front) and a jar of pickled onions (back).

A distinguishing characteristic is a pH of 4.6 or lower, which is sufficient to kill most bacteria. Pickling can preserve perishable foods for months. Antimicrobial herbs and spices, such as mustard seed, garlic, cinnamon or cloves, are often added. If the food contains sufficient moisture, a pickling brine may be produced simply by adding dry salt. For example, sauerkraut and Korean kimchi are produced by salting the vegetables to draw out excess water. Natural fermentation at room temperature, by lactic acid bacteria, produces the required acidity. Other pickles are made by placing vegetables in vinegar. Like the canning process, pickling (which includes fermentation) does not require that the food be completely sterile before it is sealed. The acidity or salinity of the solution, the temperature of fermentation, and the exclusion of oxygen determine which microorganisms dominate, and determine the flavor of the end product.

When both salt concentration and temperature are low, *Leuconostoc mesenteroides* dominates, producing a mix of acids, alcohol, and aroma compounds. At higher temperatures *Lactobacillus plantarum* dominates, which produces primarily lactic acid. Many pickles start with *Leuconostoc*, and change to *Lactobacillus* with higher acidity.

## Pickles around the World

## Central and Eastern Europe

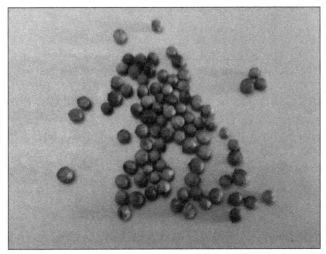

Coriander seeds are one of the spices popularly added to pickled vegetables in Europe.

In Hungary the main meal *(lunch)* usually includes some kind of pickles *(savanyúság)*, but pickles are also commonly consumed at other times of the day. The most commonly consumed pickles are sauerkraut *(savanyú káposzta)*, pickled cucumbers and peppers, and *csalamádé*, but tomatoes, carrots, beetroot, baby corn, onions, garlic, certain squashes and melons, and a few fruits like plums and apples are used to make pickles too. Stuffed pickles are specialties usually made of peppers or melons pickled after being stuffed with a cabbage filling. Pickled plum stuffed with garlic is a unique Hungarian type of pickle just like *csalamádé* and leavened cucumber *(kovászos uborka)*. *Csalamádé* is a type of mixed pickle made of cabbage, cucumber, paprika, onion, carrot, tomatoes, and bay leaf mixed up with vinegar as the fermenting agent. Leavened cucumber, unlike other types of pickled cucumbers that are around all year long, is rather a seasonal pickle produced in the summer. Cucumbers, spices, herbs, and slices of bread are put in a glass jar with salt water and kept in direct sunlight for a few days. The yeast from the bread, along with other pickling agents and spices fermented under the hot sun, give the cucumbers a unique flavor, texture, and slight carbonation. Its juice can be used instead of carbonated water to make a special type of spritzer *('Újházy fröccs')*. It is common for Hungarian households to produce their own pickles. Different regions or towns have their special recipes unique to them. Among them all the Vecsési sauerkraut *(Vecsési savanyú káposzta)* is the most famous.

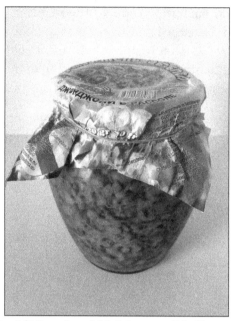

Jonjoli Georgian pickled flowers of bladdernut.

Romanian pickles (murături) are made out of beetroot, cucumbers, green tomatoes (*gogonele*), carrots, cabbage, garlic, sauerkraut (bell peppers stuffed with cabbage), bell peppers, melons, mushrooms, turnips, celery and cauliflower. Meat, like pork, can also be preserved in salt and lard.

Polish, Czech and Slovak traditional pickles are cucumbers, sauerkraut, peppers, beetroot, tomatoes, but other pickled fruits and vegetables, including plums, pumpkins and mushrooms are also common.

Russian, Ukrainian and Belarusian pickled items include beets, mushrooms, tomatoes, sauerkraut, cucumbers, ramsons, garlic, eggplant (which is typically stuffed with julienned carrots), custard squash, and watermelon. Garden produce is commonly pickled using salt, dill, blackcurrant leaves, bay leaves and garlic and is stored in a cool, dark place. The leftover brine (called *rassol* (рассол) in Russian) has a number of culinary uses in these countries, especially for cooking traditional soups, such as shchi, rassolnik, and solyanka. *Rassol*, especially cucumber or sauerkraut rassol, is also a favorite traditional remedy against morning hangover.

## Southern Europe

An Italian pickled vegetable dish is giardiniera, which includes onions, carrots, celery and cauliflower. Many places in southern Italy, particularly in Sicily, pickle eggplants and hot peppers.

In Albania, Bulgaria, Serbia, Macedonia and Turkey, mixed pickles, known as *turshi, tursija* or *turshu* form popular appetizers, which are typically eaten with *rakia*. Pickled green tomatoes, cucumbers, carrots, bell peppers, peppers, eggplants, and sauerkraut are also popular.

Turkish pickles, called *turşu*, are made out of vegetables, roots, and fruits such as peppers, cucumber, Armenian cucumber, cabbage, tomato, eggplant (aubergine), carrot, turnip, beetroot, green almond, baby watermelon, baby cantaloupe, garlic, cauliflower, bean and green plum. A mixture of spices flavor the pickles.

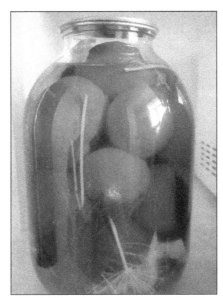

Pickled tomatoes are common in CIS.

Pickles are made out of carrots, celery, eggplants stuffed with diced carrots, cauliflower, tomatoes, and peppers.

## Northern Europe

In Britain, pickled onions and pickled eggs are often sold in pubs and fish and chip shops. Pickled beetroot, walnuts, and gherkins, and condiments such as Branston Pickle and piccalilli are typically eaten as an accompaniment to pork pies and cold meats, sandwiches or a ploughman's lunch. Other popular pickles in the UK are pickled mussels, cockles, red cabbage, mango chutney, sauerkraut, and olives. Rollmops are also quite widely available under a range of names from various producers both within and out of the UK.

Pickled herring, rollmops, and salmon are popular in Scandinavia. Pickled cucumbers and red garden beets are important as condiments for several traditional dishes. Pickled capers are also common in Scandinavian cuisine.

## United States and Canada

In the United States and Canada, pickled cucumbers (most often referred to simply as "pickles"), olives, and sauerkraut are most commonly seen, although pickles common in other nations are also available. In Canada, there may be a distinction made between gherkins (usually smaller), and pickles (larger pickled cucumbers).

Canadian pickling is similar to that of Britain. Through the winter, pickling is an important method of food preservation. Pickled cucumbers, onions, and eggs are common individual pickled foods seen in Canada. Pickled egg and pickled sausage make popular pub snacks in much of English Canada. Chow-chow is a tart vegetable mix popular in the Maritime Provinces and the Southern United States, similar to piccalilli. Pickled fish is commonly seen, as in Scotland, and kippers may be seen for breakfast, as well as plentiful smoked salmon. Meat is often also pickled or preserved in different brines throughout the winter, most prominently in the harsh climate of Newfoundland.

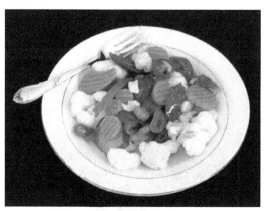

A dish of giardiniera.

In the United States, Giardiniera, a mixture of pickled peppers, celery and olives, is a popular condiment in Chicago and other cities with large Italian-American populations, and is often consumed with Italian beef sandwiches. Pickled eggs are common in the Upper Peninsula of Michigan. Pickled herring is available in the Upper Midwest. Pennsylvania Dutch Country has a strong tradition of pickled foods, including chow-chow and red beet eggs. In the Southern United States, pickled okra and watermelon rind are popular, as are deep-fried pickles and pickled pig's feet, pickled chicken eggs, pickled quail eggs, pickled garden vegetables and pickled sausage. In Mexico, chili peppers, particularly of the Jalapeño and serrano varieties, pickled with onions, carrots and herbs form common condiments. Various pickled vegetables, fish, or eggs may make a side dish to a Canadian lunch or dinner. Popular pickles in the Pacific Northwest include pickled asparagus and green beans. Pickled fruits like blueberries and early green strawberries are paired with meat dishes in restaurants.

In some parts of the United States, pickles with Kool-Aid are a popular food for children. In the United States, National Pickle Day is recognized as a food "holiday" every year on November 14.

## Mexico, Central America and South America

In the Mesoamerican region pickling is known as "encurtido" or "curtido" for short. The pickles or "curtidos" as known in Latin America are served cold, as an appetizer, as a side dish or as a tapas dish in Spain. In several Central American countries it is prepared with cabbage, onions, carrots, lemon, vinegar, oregano, and salt. In Mexico, "curtido" consists of carrots, onions, and jalapeño peppers and used to accompany meals still common in taquerias and restaurants. In order to prepare a carrot "curtido" simply add carrots to vinegar and other ingredients that are common to the region such as chilli, tomato, and onions. Varies depending on the food, in the case of sour. Another example of a type of pickling which involves the pickling of meats or seafood is the "escabeche" or "ceviches" popular in Peru, Ecuador, and throughout Latin America and the Caribbean. These dishes include the pickling of pig's feet, pig's ears, and gizzards prepared as an "escabeche" with spices and seasonings to flavor it. The ceviches consists of shrimp, octopus, and various fishes seasoned and served cold.

## Process

In traditional pickling, fruit or vegetables are submerged in brine (20-40 grams/L of salt (3.2–6.4 oz/imp gal or 2.7–5.3 oz/US gal)), or shredded and salted as in sauerkraut preparation, and held underwater by flat stones layered on top. Alternatively, a lid with an airtrap or a tight lid may be used if the lid is able to release pressure which may result from carbon dioxide buildup. Mold or (white) kahm yeast may form on the surface; kahm yeast is mostly harmless but can impart an off taste and may be removed without affecting the pickling process.

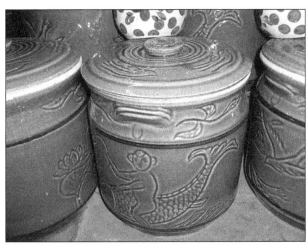

Bát Tràng porcelain vessel for pickling.

In chemical pickling, the fruits or vegetables to be pickled are placed in a sterilized jar along with brine, vinegar, or both, as well as spices, and are then allowed to mature until the desired taste is obtained.

The food can be pre-soaked in brine before transferring to vinegar. This reduces the water content of the food, which would otherwise dilute the vinegar. This method is particularly useful for fruit and vegetables with a high natural water content.

In commercial pickling, a preservative such as sodium benzoate or EDTA may also be added to enhance shelf life. In fermentation pickling, the food itself produces the preservation agent, typically by a process involving *Lactobacillus* bacteria that produce lactic acid as the preservative agent.

Alum is used in pickling to promote crisp texture and is approved as a food additive by the United States Food and Drug Administration.

"Refrigerator pickles" are unfermented pickles made by marinating fruit or vegetables in a seasoned vinegar solution. They must be stored under refrigeration or undergo canning to achieve long-term storage.

Japanese Tsukemono use a variety of pickling ingredients depending on their type , and are produced by combining these ingredients with the vegetables to be preserved and putting the mixture under pressure.

## Possible Health Hazards of Pickled Vegetables

The World Health Organization has listed pickled vegetables as a possible carcinogen, and the *British Journal of Cancer* released an online 2009 meta-analysis of research on pickles as increasing the risks of esophageal cancer. The report, citing limited data in a statistical meta analysis, indicates a potential two-fold increased risk of oesophageal cancer associated with Asian pickled vegetable consumption. Results from the research are described as having "high heterogeneity" and the study said that further well-designed prospective studies were warranted. However, their results stated "The majority of subgroup analyses showed a statistically significant association between consuming pickled vegetables and Oesophageal Squamous Cell Carcinoma".

The 2009 meta-analysis reported heavy infestation of pickled vegetables with fungi. Some common fungi can facilitate the formation of N-nitroso compounds, which are strong oesophageal carcinogens in several animal models. Roussin red methyl ester, a non-alkylating nitroso compound with tumour-promoting effect in vitro, was identified in pickles from Linxian in much higher concentrations than in samples from low-incidence areas. Fumonisin mycotoxins have been shown to cause liver and kidney tumours in rodents.

A 2017 study in *Chinese Journal of Cancer* has linked salted vegetables (common among Chinese cuisine) to a fourfold increase in nasopharynx cancer, where fermentation was a critical step in creating nitrosamines, which some are confirmed carcinogens, as well as activation of Epstein–Barr virus by fermentation products.

Historically, pickling caused health concerns for reasons associated with copper salts, as explained in the mid-19th century *The English and Australian Cookery Book*: "The evidence of the Lancet commissioner (Dr. Hassall) and Mr. Blackwell (of the eminent firm of Crosse and Blackwell) went to prove that the pickles sold in the shops are nearly always artificially colored, and are thus rendered highly unwholesome, if not actually poisonous."

# Curing

Curing is any of various food preservation and flavoring processes of foods such as meat, fish and vegetables, by the addition of salt, with the aim of drawing moisture out of the food by the process of osmosis. Because curing increases the solute concentration in the food and hence decreases its water potential, the food becomes inhospitable for the microbe growth that causes food spoilage. Curing can be traced back to antiquity, and was the primary way of preserving meat and fish until the late-19th century. Dehydration was the earliest form of food curing. Many curing processes also involve smoking, spicing, cooking, or the addition of combinations of sugar, nitrate, nitrite.

Meat preservation in general (of meat from livestock, game, and poultry) comprises the set of all treatment processes for preserving the properties, taste, texture, and color of raw, partially cooked, or cooked meats while keeping them edible and safe to consume. Curing has been the dominant method of meat preservation for thousands of years, although modern developments like refrigeration and synthetic preservatives have begun to complement and supplant it.

While meat-preservation processes like curing were mainly developed in order to prevent disease and to increase food security, the advent of modern preservation methods mean that in most developed countries today curing is instead mainly practised for its cultural value and desirable impact on the texture and taste of food. For lesser-developed countries, curing remains a key process in the production, transport and availability of meat.

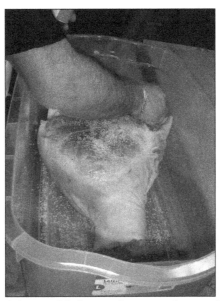

Sea salt being added to raw ham to make prosciutto.

Some traditional cured meat (such as authentic Parma ham and some authentic Spanish chorizo and Italian salami,) are cured with salt alone. Today, potassium nitrate and sodium nitrite (in conjunction with salt) are the most common agents in curing meat, because they bond to the myoglobin and act as a substitute for the oxygen, thus turning myoglobin red. More recent evidence shows that these chemicals also inhibit the growth of the bacteria that cause the disease botulism. The combination of table salt with nitrates or nitrites, called curing salt, is often dyed pink to distinguish it from table salt. Neither table salt, nor any of the nitrites or nitrates commonly used in curing (e.g. sodium nitrate, sodium nitrite, and potassium nitrate) is naturally pink.

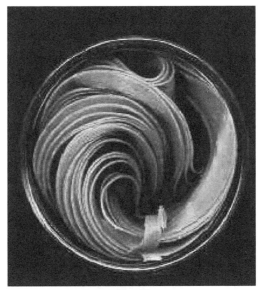

Slices of beef in a can.

## Necessity of Curing

Untreated meat decomposes rapidly if it is not preserved, at a speed that depends on several factors, including ambient humidity, temperature, and the presence of pathogens. Most meats cannot be kept at room temperature in excess of a few days without spoiling.

If kept in excess of this time, meat begins to change color and exude a foul odor, indicating the decomposition of the food. Ingestion of such spoiled meat can cause serious food poisonings, like botulism. Salt-curing processes have been developed since antiquity in order to ensure food safety without relying on artificial anti-bacterial agents.

While the short shelf life of fresh meat does not pose a significant problem when access to it is easy and supply is abundant, in times of scarcity and famine, or when the meat must be carried over long voyages, it spoils very quickly. In such circumstances the usefulness of preserving foods containing nutritional value for transport and storage is obvious.

Curing can significantly extend the life of meat before it spoils, by making it inhospitable to the growth of spoilage microbes.

## Chemical Actions

### Salt

Salt (sodium chloride) is the primary ingredient used in meat curing. Removal of water and addition of salt to meat creates a solute-rich environment where osmotic pressure draws water out of micro-organisms, slowing down their growth. Doing this requires a concentration of salt of nearly 20%. In addition, salt causes the soluble proteins to come to the surface of the meat that was used to make the sausages. These proteins coagulate when the sausage is heated, helping to hold the sausage together.

### Sugar

The sugar added to meat for the purpose of curing it comes in many forms, including honey, corn syrup solids, and maple syrup. However, with the exception of bacon, it does not contribute much to the flavor, but it does alleviate the harsh flavor of the salt. Sugar also contributes to the growth of beneficial bacteria such as *Lactobacillus* by feeding them.

### Nitrates and Nitrites

Nitrates and nitrites not only help kill bacteria, but also produce a characteristic flavor and give meat a pink or red color. Nitrite (($NO_2^-$)) is generally supplied by sodium nitrite or (indirectly) by potassium nitrate. Nitrite salts are most often used in curing. Nitrate is specifically used only in a few curing conditions and products where nitrite (which may be generated from nitrate) must be generated in the product over long periods of time.

Nitrite further breaks down in the meat into nitric oxide (NO), which then binds to the iron atom in the center of myoglobin's heme group, reducing oxidation and causing a reddish-brown color (nitrosomyoglobin) when raw and the characteristic cooked-ham pink color (nitrosohemochrome or nitrosyl-heme) when cooked. The addition of ascorbate to cured meat reduces formation of nitrosamines, but increases the nitrosylation of iron.

The use of nitrite and nitrate salts for meat in the US has been formally used since 1925. Because of the relatively high toxicity of nitrite (the lethal dose in humans is about 22 mg/kg of body weight), the maximum allowed nitrite concentration in meat products is 200 ppm. Plasma nitrite is reduced in persons with endothelial dysfunction.

Nitrosyl-heme.

The use of nitrites in food preservation is controversial due to the potential for the formation of nitrosamines when nitrites are present in high concentrations and the product is cooked at high temperatures. The effect is seen for red or processed meat, but not for white meat or fish. Nitrates and nitrites may cause cancer and the production of carcinogenic nitrosamines can be potently inhibited by the use of the antioxidants Vitamin C and the alpha-tocopherol form of Vitamin E during curing. Under simulated gastric conditions, nitrosothiols rather than nitrosamines are the main nitroso species being formed. The use of either compound is therefore regulated; for example, in the United States, the concentration of nitrates and nitrites is generally limited to 200 ppm or lower. While the meat industry considers them irreplaceable because of their low cost and efficacy at maintaining color, botulism is an extremely rare disease (less than 1000 cases reported worldwide per year), and almost always associated with home preparations of food storing. Furthermore, while the FDA has set a limit of 200 ppm of nitrates for cured meat, they are not allowed and not recognized as safe in most other foods, even foods that are not cooked at high temperatures, such as cheese.

## Nitrites from Celery

Processed meats without "added nitrites" may be misleading as they may be using naturally occurring nitrites from celery instead.

A 2019 report from Consumer Reports found that using celery (or other natural sources) as a curing agent introduced naturally occurring nitrates and nitrites. The USDA allows the term "uncured" or "no nitrates or nitrites added" on products using these natural sources of nitrites, which provides the consumer a false sense of making a healthier choice. The Consumer Reports investigation also provides the average level of sodium, nitrates and nitrites found per gram of meat in their report.

Consumer Reports and the Center for Science in the Public Interest filed a formal request to the USDA to change the labeling requirements this year.

## Smoke

Meat can also be preserved by "smoking". If the smoke is hot enough to slow-cook the meat, this will also keep it tender. One method of smoking calls for a smokehouse with damp wood chips or sawdust. In North America, hardwoods such as hickory, mesquite, and maple are commonly used for smoking, as are the wood from fruit trees such as apple, cherry, and plum, and even corncobs.

Smoking helps seal the outer layer of the food being cured, making it more difficult for bacteria to enter. It can be done in combination with other curing methods such as salting. Common smoking styles include hot smoking, smoke roasting (pit barbecuing) and cold smoking. Smoke roasting and hot smoking cook the meat while cold smoking does not. If the meat is cold smoked, it should be dried quickly to limit bacterial growth during the critical period where the meat is not yet dry. This can be achieved, as with jerky, by slicing the meat thinly.

The smoking of food directly with wood smoke is known to contaminate the food with carcinogenic polycyclic aromatic hydrocarbons.

## Effect of Meat Preservation

## On Health

Since the 20th century, with respect to the relationship between diet and human disease (e.g. cardiovascular, etc.), scientists have conducted studies on the effects of lipolysis on vacuum-packed or frozen meat. In particular, by analyzing entrecôtes of frozen beef during 270 days at −20 °C (−4 °F), scientists found an important phospholipase that accompanies the loss of some unsaturated fat n-3 and n-6, which are already low in the flesh of ruminants.

In 2015, the International Agency for Research on Cancer of the World Health Organization classified processed meat, that is, meat that has undergone salting, curing, fermenting, or smoking, as "carcinogenic to humans".

## On Trade

The improvement of methods of meat preservation, and of the means of transport of preserved products, has notably permitted the separation of areas of production and areas of consumption, which can now be distant without it posing a problem, permitting the exportation of meats.

For example, the appearance in the 1980s of preservation techniques under controlled atmosphere sparked a small revolution in the world's market for sheep meat: the lamb of New Zealand, one of the world's largest exporters of lamb, could henceforth be sold as fresh meat, since it could be preserved from 12 to 16 weeks, which would be a sufficient duration for it to reach Europe by boat. Before, meat from New Zealand was frozen, thus had a much lower value on European shelves. With the arrival of the new "chilled" meats, New Zealand could compete even more strongly with local producers of fresh meat. The use of controlled atmosphere to avoid the depreciation which affects frozen meat is equally useful in other meat markets, such as that for pork, which now also enjoys an international trade.

# Salting

Salting is the preservation of food with dry edible salt. It is related to pickling in general and more specifically to brining (preparing food with brine, that is, salty water) and is one form of curing. It is one of the oldest methods of preserving food, and two historically significant salt-cured foods are salted fish (usually dried and salted cod or salted herring) and salt-cured meat (such as bacon). Vegetables such as runner beans and cabbage are also often preserved in this manner.

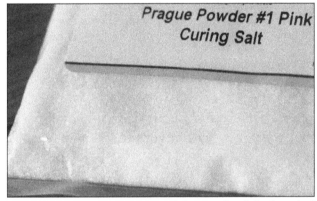

Bag of Prague powder 1, also known as "curing salt" or "pink salt." It's typically a combination of salt and sodium nitrite, with the pink color added to distinguish it from ordinary salt.

Salting is used because most bacteria, fungi and other potentially pathogenic organisms cannot survive in a highly salty environment, due to the hypertonic nature of salt. Any living cell in such an environment will become dehydrated through osmosis and die or become temporarily inactivated.

It was discovered in the 19th century that salt mixed with nitrates (saltpeter) would color meats red, rather than grey, and consumers at that time then strongly preferred the red-colored meat. The food hence preserved stays healthy and fresh for days avoiding bacterial decay.

# Fruit Preserves

Fruit preserves are preparations of fruits, vegetables and sugar, often stored in glass jam jars and Mason jars.

Many varieties of fruit preserves are made globally, including sweet fruit preserves, such as those made from strawberry or apricot, and savory preserves, such as those made from tomatoes or squash. The ingredients used and how they are prepared determine the type of preserves; jams, jellies, and marmalades are all examples of different styles of fruit preserves that vary based upon the fruit used. In English, the word, in plural form, "preserves" is used to describe all types of jams and jellies.

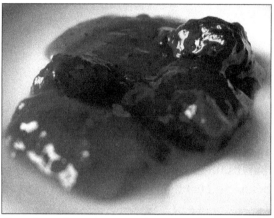

Strawberry jam, one type of common fruit preserve.

## Variations

### Chutney

A chutney is a relish of Indian origin made of fruit, spices and herbs. Although originally intended to be eaten soon after production, modern chutneys are often made to be sold, so require preservatives – often sugar and vinegar – to ensure they have a suitable shelf life. Mango chutney, for example, is mangoes reduced with sugar.

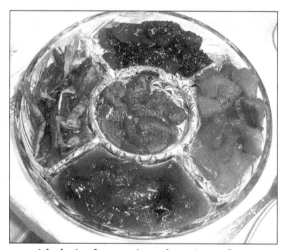

Five varieties of fruit preserves (clockwise from top): apple, quince, plum, squash, orange (in the center).

### Confit

While confit, the past participle of the French verb *confire*, "to preserve", is most often applied to preservation of meats, it is also used for fruits or vegetables seasoned and cooked with honey or sugar till jam-like. Savory confits, such as ones made with garlic or fennel, may call for a savory oil, such as virgin olive oil, as the preserving agent.

Konfyt (Afrikaans: "jam" or "fruit preserve") is a type of jam eaten in Southern Africa. It is made by boiling selected fruit or fruits (such as strawberries, apricots, oranges, lemons, water melons, berries, peaches, prickly pears or others) and sugar, and optionally adding a small quantity of ginger to enhance the flavor. The origins of the jam is obscure but it is theorized that it came from the French. The word is also based on the French term *confiture* via the Dutch *confijt* (meaning candied fruit).

## Conserve

A conserve, or whole fruit jam, is a preserve made of fruit stewed in sugar. Traditional whole fruit preserves are particularly popular in Eastern Europe (Russia, Ukraine, Belarus) where they are called varenye, the Baltic region where they're known by a native name in each of the countries (Lithuanian: *uogienė*, Latvian: *ievārījums*, Estonian: *moos*, Romanian: *dulceață*), as well as in many regions of Western, Central and Southern Asia, where they are referred to as murabba.

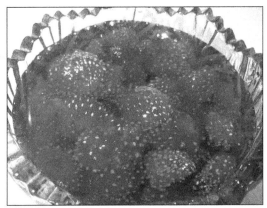
Strawberry varenye (murabba).

Often the making of conserves can be trickier than making a standard jam; it requires cooking or sometimes steeping in the hot sugar mixture for just enough time to allow the flavor to be extracted from the fruit, and sugar to penetrate the fruit; and not cooking too long such that the fruit will break down and liquify. This process can also be achieved by spreading the dry sugar over raw fruit in layers, and leaving for several hours to steep into the fruit, then just heating the resulting mixture only to bring to the setting point. As a result of this minimal cooking, some fruits are not particularly suitable for making into conserves, because they require cooking for longer periods to avoid issues such as tough skins. Currants and gooseberries, and a number of plums are among these fruits.

Because of this shorter cooking period, not as much pectin will be released from the fruit, and as such, conserves (particularly home-made conserves) will sometimes be slightly softer set than some jams.

An alternative definition holds that conserves are preserves made from a mixture of fruits or vegetables. Conserves may also include dried fruit or nuts.

## Fruit Butter

Fruit butter, in this context, refers to a process where the whole fruit is forced through a sieve or blended after the heating process.

Fruit butters are generally made from larger fruits, such as apples, plums, peaches or grapes. Cook until softened and run through a sieve to give a smooth consistency. After sieving, cook the pulp add sugar and cook as rapidly as possible with constant stirring. The finished product should mound up when dropped from a spoon, but should not cut like jelly. Neither should there be any free liquid.

## Fruit Curd

Fruit curd is a dessert topping and spread usually made with lemon, lime, orange, or raspberry. The basic ingredients are beaten egg yolks, sugar, fruit juice and zest which are gently cooked together until thick and then allowed to cool, forming a soft, smooth, intensely flavored spread. Some recipes also include egg whites or butter.

## Fruit Spread

Although the FDA has *Requirements for Specific Standardized Fruit Butters, Jellies, Preserves, and Related Products*, there is no specification of the meaning of the term fruit spread. Although some assert it refers to a jam or preserve with no added sugar, there are many "fruit spreads" by leading manufacturers that do contain added sugar. This can be easily verified by searching the listings under *fruit spread* on common web sites, such as those of Amazon or Walmart, or to look at the ingredient list and nutritional information on specific fruit spread products.

## Jam

Jam typically contains both the juice and flesh of a fruit or vegetable, although one cookbook defines it as a cooked and jelled puree. The term "jam" refers to a product made of whole fruit cut into pieces or crushed, then heated with water and sugar to activate its pectin before being put into containers:

Berolzheimer's opinion is that "Jams are usually made from pulp and juice of one fruit, rather than a combination of several fruits. Berries and other small fruits are most frequently used, though larger fruits such as apricots, peaches, or plums cut into small pieces or crushed are also used for jams. Good jam has a soft even consistency without distinct pieces of fruit, a bright color, a good fruit flavor and a semi-jellied texture that is easy to spread but has no free liquid."

Pectin is mainly D-galacturonic acid connected by $\alpha$ (1–4) glycosidic linkages. The side chains of pectin may contain small amounts of other sugars such as L-fructose, D-glucose, D-mannose, and D-xylose. In jams, pectin is what thickens the final product via cross-linking of the large polymer chains.

*Freezer jam* is uncooked (or cooked less than 5 minutes), then stored frozen. It is popular in parts of North America for its very fresh taste.

Recipes without added pectin use the natural pectin in the fruit to set. Tart apples, sour blackberries, cranberries, currants, gooseberries, Concord grapes, soft plums, and quinces work well in recipes without added pectin.

Other fruits, such as apricots, blueberries, cherries, peaches, pineapple, raspberries, rhubarb, and strawberries are low in pectin. In order to set, or gel, they must be combined with one of the higher pectin fruits or used with commercially produced or homemade pectin. Use of added pectin decreases cooking time.

In Canada, fruit jam is categorized into two types: fruit jam and fruit jam with pectin. Both types contain fruit, fruit pulp or canned fruit and are boiled with water and a sweetening ingredient. Both must have 66% water-soluble solids. Fruit jam and fruit jam with pectin may contain a class II preservative, a pH adjusting agent or an antifoaming agent. Both types cannot contain apple or rhubarb fruit.

Though both types of jam are very similar, there are some differences in fruit percent, added pectin and added acidity. Fruit jam must have at least 45% fruit and may contain added pectin to compensate for the natural pectin level found in the fruit. Fruit jam with pectin need only contain 27% fruit and is allowed to contain added acidity to compensate for the natural acidity of the fruit.

Jam is created by boiling fruit, fruit pulp or canned fruit with water to and adding a sweetening ingredient. In Canada, jam must contain at least 45% of the named fruit and 66% water soluble solids. Jam may contain small amounts of pectin, pectinous preparation or acid ingredients if there is a deficiency in natural pectin. In Canada, Jam may also contain a class II preservative, a pH adjusting agent, an antifoaming agent and cannot contain any apple or rhubarb.

## Jelly

This drawing depicts a pectin molecule. These molecules combine to form the network responsible for making jelly.

In North America, jelly (from the French *gelée*) refers exclusively to a clear or translucent fruit spread made from sweetened fruit (or vegetable) juice—thus differing from jam by excluding the fruit's flesh—and is set by using its naturally occurring pectin, whereas outside North America jelly more often refers to a gelatin-based dessert, though the term is also used to refer to clear jams such as blackcurrant and apple. In the United Kingdom, redcurrant jelly is a condiment often served with lamb, game meat including venison, turkey and goose in a festive or Sunday roast. It is a clear jam, set with pectin from the fruit, and is made in the same way, by adding the redcurrants to sugar, boiling, and straining.

Pectin is essential to the formation of jelly because it acts as a gelling agent, meaning when the pectin chains combine, they create a network that results in a gel. The strength and effectiveness of the side chains and the bonds they form depend on the pH of the pectin, the optimal pH is between 2.8 and 3.2.

Additional pectin may be added where the original fruit does not supply enough, for example with grapes. Jelly can be made from sweet, savory or hot ingredients. It is made by a process similar to that used for making jam, with the additional step of filtering out the fruit pulp after the initial heating. A muslin or stockinette "jelly bag" is traditionally used as a filter, suspended by string over a bowl to allow the straining to occur gently under gravity. It is important not to attempt to force the straining process, for example by squeezing the mass of fruit in the muslin, or the clarity of the resulting jelly will be compromised. Jelly can come in a variety of flavors such as grape jelly, strawberry jelly, hot chile pepper, and others. It is typically eaten with a variety of foods. This includes jelly with toast, or a peanut butter and jelly sandwich.

Good jelly is clear and sparkling and has a fresh flavor of the fruit from which it is made. It is tender enough to quiver when moved, but holds angles when cut. Pectin is best extracted from the fruit by heat, therefore cook the fruit until soft before straining to obtain the juice . Pour cooked fruit into a jelly bag which has been wrung out of cold water. Hang up and let drain. When dripping has ceased the bag may be squeezed to remove remaining juice, but this may cause cloudy jelly.

In Canada, the Food and Drug Regulations of the Food and Drugs Act of Canada categorizes jelly into two types: jelly, and jelly with pectin. Jelly may be made from the fruit, the fruit juice, or a fruit juice concentrate, and must contain at least 62% water soluble solids. Jelly may contain an acid ingredient that makes up for any lack in the natural acidity of the fruit, a chemical to adjust the pH, and/or an antifoaming agent. Jelly with pectin must be made with a minimum of 62% water soluble solids and a minimum of 32% juice of the named fruit, and may contain an acid ingredient that compensates for the lack in the natural acidity of the fruit; the additional juice of another fruit; a gelling agent; food color; a Class II preservative (such as benzoates, sorbates, or nitrites); a chemical to adjust the pH; and/or an antifoaming agent.

## Marmalade

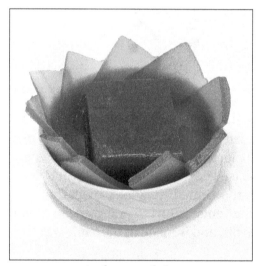

Apple marmalade.

Marmalade is a fruit preserve made from the juice and peel of citrus fruits boiled with sugar and water. It can be produced from lemons, limes, grapefruits, mandarins, sweet oranges, bergamots and other citrus fruits, or any combination thereof. Marmalade is generally distinguished from jam by its fruit peel.

The benchmark citrus fruit for marmalade production in Britain is the Spanish Seville orange,

*Citrus aurantium* var. *aurantium*, prized for its high pectin content, which gives a good set. The peel has a distinctive bitter taste which it imparts to the preserve. In America, marmalade is sweet.

## Production

In general, jam is produced by taking mashed or chopped fruit or vegetable pulp and boiling it with sugar and water. The proportion of sugar and fruit varies according to the type of fruit and its ripeness, but a rough starting point is equal weights of each. When the mixture reaches a temperature of 104 °C (219 °F), the acid and the pectin in the fruit react with the sugar, and the jam will set on cooling. However, most cooks work by trial and error, bringing the mixture to a "fast rolling boil", watching to see if the seething mass changes texture, and dropping small samples on a plate to see if they run or set.

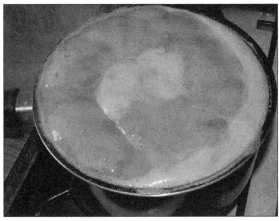
Jam being made in a pot.

Commercially produced jams are usually produced using one of two methods. The first is the open pan method, which is essentially a larger scale version of the method a home jam maker would use. This gives a traditional flavor, with some caramelization of the sugars. The second commercial process involves the use of a vacuum vessel, where the jam is placed under a vacuum, which has the effect of reducing its boiling temperature to anywhere between 65 and 80 °C depending on the recipe and the end result desired. The lower boiling temperature enables the water to be driven off as it would be when using the traditional open pan method, but with the added benefit of retaining more of the volatile flavor compounds from the fruit, preventing caramelization of the sugars, and of course reducing the overall energy required to make the product. However, once the desired amount of water has been driven off, the jam still needs to be heated briefly to 95 to 100 °C (203 to 212 °F) to kill off any micro-organisms that may be present; the vacuum pan method does not kill them all.

During commercial filling it is common to use a flame to sterilize the rim and lid of jars to destroy any yeasts and molds which may cause spoilage during storage. Steam is commonly injected immediately prior to lidding to create a vacuum, which both helps prevent spoilage and pulls down tamper-evident safety button when used.

## Packaging

Glass or plastic jars are an efficient method of storing and preserving jam. Though sugar can keep for exceedingly long times, containing it in a jar is far more useful than older methods. Other methods of packaging jam, especially for industrially produced products, include cans and plastic packets, especially used in the food service industry for individual servings. Fruit preserves typically are of low water activity and can be stored at room temperature after opening, if used within a short period of time.

# Canning

Canning is a method of preserving food in which the food contents are processed and sealed in an airtight container (jars like Mason jars, and steel and tin cans). Canning provides a shelf life typically ranging from one to five years, although under specific circumstances it can be much longer. A freeze-dried canned product, such as canned dried lentils, could last as long as 30 years in an edible state. In 1974, samples of canned food from the wreck of the *Bertrand*, a steamboat that sank in the Missouri River in 1865, were tested by the National Food Processors Association. Although appearance, smell and vitamin content had deteriorated, there was no trace of microbial growth and the 109-year-old food was determined to be still safe to eat.

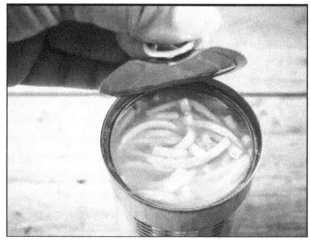

Canned soup.

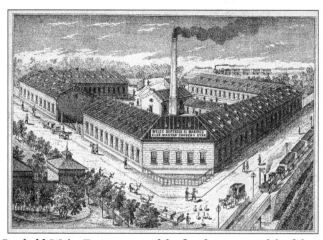

The Berthold-Weiss Factory, one of the first large canned food factories.

## Methods

The original fragile and heavy glass containers presented challenges for transportation, and glass jars were largely replaced in commercial canneries with cylindrical tin can or wrought-iron canisters (later shortened to "cans") following the work of Peter Durand (1810). Cans are cheaper and quicker to make, and much less fragile than glass jars. Glass jars have remained popular for some high-value products and in home canning. Can openers were not invented for another thirty years — at first, soldiers had to cut the cans open with bayonets or smash them open with rocks. Today, tin-coated steel is the material most commonly used. Laminate vacuum pouches are also used for canning, such as used in MREs and Capri Sun drinks.

To prevent the food from being spoiled before and during containment, a number of methods are used: pasteurisation, boiling (and other applications of high temperature over a period of time), refrigeration, freezing, drying, vacuum treatment, antimicrobial agents that are natural to the recipe of the foods being preserved, a sufficient dose of ionizing radiation, submersion in a strong saline solution, acid, base, osmotically extreme (for example very sugary) or other microbially-challenging environments.

Other than sterilization, no method is perfectly dependable as a preservative. For example, the microorganism *Clostridium botulinum* (which causes botulism) can be eliminated only at temperatures above the boiling point of water.

From a public safety point of view, foods with low acidity (a pH more than 4.6) need sterilization under high temperature (116–130 °C). To achieve temperatures above the boiling point requires the use of a pressure canner. Foods that must be pressure canned include most vegetables, meat, seafood, poultry, and dairy products. The only foods that may be safely canned in an ordinary boiling water bath are highly acidic ones with a pH below 4.6, such as fruits, pickled vegetables, or other foods to which acidic additives have been added.

## Double Seams

Invented in 1888 by Max Ams, modern double seams provide an airtight seal to the tin can. This airtight nature is crucial to keeping micro-organisms out of the can and keeping its contents sealed inside. Thus, double seamed cans are also known as Sanitary Cans. Developed in 1900 in Europe, this sort of can was made of the traditional cylindrical body made with tin plate. The two ends (lids) were attached using what is now called a double seam. A can thus sealed is impervious to contamination by creating two tight continuous folds between the can's cylindrical body and the lids. This eliminated the need for solder and allowed improvements in manufacturing speed, reducing cost.

Double seaming uses rollers to shape the can, lid and the final double seam. To make a sanitary can and lid suitable for double seaming, manufacture begins with a sheet of coated tin plate. To create the can body, rectangles are cut and curled around a die, and welded together creating a cylinder with a side seam.

Rollers are then used to flare out one or both ends of the cylinder to create a quarter circle flange around the circumference. Precision is required to ensure that the welded sides are perfectly aligned, as any misalignment will cause inconsistent flange shape, compromising its integrity.

A circle is then cut from the sheet using a die cutter. The circle is shaped in a stamping press to create a downward countersink to fit snugly into the can body. The result can be compared to an upside down and very flat top hat. The outer edge is then curled down and around about 140 degrees using rollers to create the end curl.

The result is a steel tube with a flanged edge, and a countersunk steel disc with a curled edge. A rubber compound is put inside the curl.

## Seaming

The body and end are brought together in a seamer and held in place by the base plate and chuck, respectively. The base plate provides a sure footing for the can body during the seaming operation and the chuck fits snugly into the end (lid). The result is the countersink of the end sits inside the top of the can body just below the flange. The end curl protrudes slightly beyond the flange.

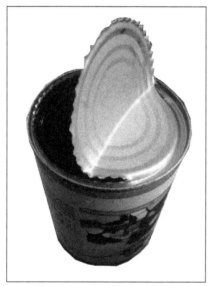

Opened can.

## First Operation

Once brought together in the seamer, the seaming head presses a first operation roller against the end curl. The end curl is pressed against the flange curling it in toward the body and under the flange. The flange is also bent downward, and the end and body are now loosely joined together. The first operation roller is then retracted. At this point five thicknesses of steel exist in the seam. From the outside in they are:

- End,

- Flange,

- End Curl,

- Body,

- Countersink.

## Second Operation

The seaming head then engages the second operation roller against the partly formed seam. The second operation presses all five steel components together tightly to form the final seal. The five layers in the final seam are then called; a) End, b) Body Hook, c) Cover Hook, d) Body, e) Countersink. All sanitary cans require a filling medium within the seam because otherwise the metal-to-metal contact will not maintain a hermetic seal. In most cases, a rubberized compound is placed inside the end curl radius, forming the critical seal between the end and the body.

Probably the most important innovation since the introduction of double seams is the welded side seam. Prior to the welded side seam, the can body was folded and/or soldered together, leaving a relatively thick side seam. The thick side seam required that the side seam end juncture at the end curl to have more metal to curl around before closing in behind the Body Hook or flange, with a greater opportunity for error.

## Seamer Setup and Quality Assurance

Many different parts during the seaming process are critical in ensuring that a can is airtight and vacuum sealed. The dangers of a can that is not hermetically sealed are contamination by foreign objects (bacteria or fungicide sprays), or that the can could leak or spoil.

One important part is the seamer setup. This process is usually performed by an experienced technician. Amongst the parts that need setup are seamer rolls and chucks which have to be set in their exact position (using a feeler gauge or a clearance gauge). The lifter pressure and position, roll and chuck designs, tooling wear, and bearing wear all contribute to a good double seam.

Incorrect setups can be non-intuitive. For example, due to the springback effect, a seam can appear loose, when in reality it was closed too tight and has opened up like a spring. For this reason, experienced operators and good seamer setup are critical to ensure that double seams are properly closed.

Quality control usually involves taking full cans from the line – one per seamer head, at least once or twice per shift, and performing a teardown operation (wrinkle/tightness), mechanical tests (external thickness, seamer length/height and countersink) as well as cutting the seam open with a twin blade saw and measuring with a double seam inspection system. The combination of these measurements will determine the seam's quality.

Use of a statistical process control (SPC) software in conjunction with a manual double-seam monitor, computerized double seam scanner, or even a fully automatic double seam inspection system makes the laborious process of double seam inspection faster and much more accurate. Statistically tracking the performance of each head or seaming station of the can seamer allows for better prediction of can seamer issues, and may be used to plan maintenance when convenient, rather than to simply react after bad or unsafe cans have been produced.

## Nutritional Value

Canning is a way of processing food to extend its shelf life. The idea is to make food available and edible long after the processing time. A 1997 study found that canned fruits and vegetables are as rich with dietary fiber and vitamins as the same corresponding fresh or frozen foods, and in some cases the canned products are richer than their fresh or frozen counterparts. The heating process during canning appears to make dietary fiber more soluble, and therefore more readily fermented in the colon into gases and physiologically active byproducts. Canned tomatoes have a higher available lycopene content. Consequently, canned meat and vegetables are often among the list of food items that are stocked during emergencies.

## Potential Hazards

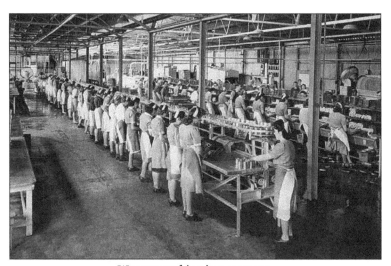
Women working in a cannery.

In the beginning of the 19th century the process of canning foods was mainly done by small canneries. These canneries were full of overlooked sanitation problems, such as poor hygiene and unsanitary work environments. Since the refrigerator did not exist and industrial canning standards were not set in place it was very common for contaminated cans to slip onto the grocery store shelves.

## Migration of Can Components

In canning toxicology, *migration* is the movement of substances from the can itself into the contents. Potential toxic substances that can migrate are lead, causing lead poisoning, or bisphenol A (BPA), a potential endocrine disruptor that is an ingredient in the epoxy commonly used to coat the inner surface of cans. Some cans are manufactured with a BPA-free enamel lining produced from plant oils and resins. On 20 February 2018, *Packaging Digest* reported that "At least 90%" of food cans no longer contained BPA.

## Salt (Sodium Chloride)

Salt (sodium chloride), dissolved in water, is used in the canning process. As a result, canned food can be a major source of dietary salt. Too much salt increases the risk of health problems, including high blood pressure. Therefore, health authorities have recommended limitations of dietary sodium. Many canned products are available in low-salt and no-salt alternatives.

Rinsing thoroughly after opening may reduce the amount of salt in canned foods, since much of the salt content is thought to be in the liquid, rather than the food itself.

## Botulism

Foodborne botulism results from contaminated foodstuffs in which *C. botulinum* spores have been allowed to germinate and produce botulism toxin, and this typically occurs in canned non-acidic food substances that have not received a strong enough thermal heat treatment. *C. botulinum* prefers low oxygen environments and is a poor competitor to other bacteria, but its spores are resistant to thermal treatments. When a canned food is sterilized insufficiently, most other bacteria besides the *C. botulinum* spores are killed, and the spores can germinate and produce botulism toxin. Botulism is a rare but serious paralytic illness, leading to paralysis that typically starts with the muscles of the face and then spreads towards the limbs. The botulinum toxin is extremely dangerous because it cannot be detected by sight or smell, and ingestion of even a small amount of the toxin can be deadly. In severe forms, it leads to paralysis of the breathing muscles and causes respiratory failure. In view of this life-threatening complication, all suspected cases of botulism are treated as medical emergencies, and public health officials are usually involved to prevent further cases from the same source.

## Canning and Economic Recession

Canned goods and canning supplies sell particularly well in times of recession due to the tendency of financially stressed individuals to engage in cocooning, a term used by retail analysts to describe the phenomenon in which people choose to stay at home instead of adding expenditures to their budget by dining out and socializing outside the home.

In February 2009 during a recession, the United States saw an 11.5% rise in sales of canning-related items.

Some communities in the US have county canning centers which are available for teaching canning, or shared community kitchens which can be rented for canning one's own foods.

## Food Drying

Food drying is one of the oldest methods of preserving food. Since drying reduces the moisture in foods making them lightweight and convenient to store, it can easily be used in place of other food preservation techniques. In fact, one can even use drying along with other food preservation techniques such as freezing or canning, which would make the process of food preservation even better.

 Drying food is simple, safe and easy to learn. The early American settlers practiced drying food using the natural forces of sun and wind and today, the use of technology has revolutionized this method of preserving food. With modern food dehydrators, foods such as fruit leathers, fruit chips, dried nuts and seeds and meat jerky, can all be dried year-round at home.

Being easy to store and carry and requiring no refrigeration makes dried foods ideal for domestic use as well as for use in the rough outdoors.

Moreover, dried foods are good sources of quick energy and wholesome nutrition, since the only thing lost during preservation is moisture. For instance, meat jerky, dried nuts and seeds are good sources of protein for a snack or a meal. The fruit leathers and chips provide plenty of quick energy. Dried vegetables, too, can be used to prepare wholesome casseroles and soups and the nutritional value can be enhanced by using the soaking water for cooking. Therefore, dried foods are an easy food option for busy executives, hungry backpackers and active women and children, all of whom can benefit from the ease of use and nutritional content of dried foods.

## How Drying Preserves Food

Drying basically dehydrates or removes the moisture from the food and this simple action inhibits the growth of bacteria, mold and yeast. Moreover, it slows down the enzyme action without de-activating them. These factors ensure that food does not spoil easily and hence, makes drying an effective food preservation technique.

Since drying removes the water from the food, the weight of the food item also reduces. This not only makes it lighter but also shrinks it in size. In order to use the food, all one has to do is add water to it.

The best temperature to dry foods and preserve them is 140 °F. However, for meats and poultry, the USDA Meat and Poultry Hotline recommends heating meat to 160 °F and poultry to 165 °F before starting the drying process. Once the heating is done, the dehydrator temperature should be consistent at 130 to 140 °F. Using temperatures higher than this will result in cooking the food instead of drying it. The food will cook on the outside and the moisture will remain trapped within. Drying is a slow process and one shouldn't try and speed it up by raising the temperature.

Another factor that helps with drying food is humidity. Since drying involves extracting the moisture from the food items and expelling it into the surrounding air, low humidity will help with the drying process. If the humidity is high, drying will be slower simply because the surrounding air would also be laden with moisture. By increasing the currents or flow of air, one can speed up the drying process.

There are several ways of drying foods – in the sun, in an oven or in a commercial dehydrator. However, in either case, it is important to have the right temperature, air flow and level of humidity.

## Drying Foods Out-of-doors

## Sun Drying

Drying food in the sun is a safe and economical way to preserve food, especially fruits. Meats and vegetables, however, cannot be dried outdoors since they have a low sugar and acid content. Fruits have a high sugar and acid content, which makes sun drying safe and easy. Meats and vegetables are best dried indoors in a controlled oven or dehydrator since temperature and humidity are essential when preserving these food groups.

In order to dry food in the sun, one needs to have both warm temperatures and a constant breeze. A minimum temperature of 85 °F is essential while higher temperatures are obviously better. The high temperature will extract the moisture while the breeze would help to dispel it into the surrounding air. A low level of humidity is also essential for successful sun drying. The high humidity levels in the South make sun drying difficult. Humidity of below 60 percent is ideal.

Raisins dried in the sun are probably the most widely known of dried fruits. The sunny region of California produces a large portion of these raisins and the reason is simple. The temperatures in the San Joaquin valley are warm, the humidity is low and there is a constant breeze. These conditions are ideal for drying and preserving fruits, especially grapes.

Sun drying is a slow and time-consuming process since the unpredictable and uncontrollable weather is the drying agent. Moreover, it is this unpredictability that also makes sun drying a risky process. For instance, in California, sudden rains can ruin the entire supply of raisins. Not only that, having the ideal mix of temperature, humidity and air flow is often difficult to achieve and this prompts one to look for other methods of drying food.

Fruit that is being dried in the sun needs to be protected from the cool night air that could add the moisture back to the fruit. Therefore, the fruits must either be brought in every night or put under some form of shelter to protect them from the night dew.

## Equipment

For drying food in the sun, one needs racks or screens that are placed on blocks or on a concrete surface. This arrangement and equipment ensures adequate flow of air around the food. To prevent transfer of moisture from the earth, place the racks or screens on a concrete surface or over a sheet of aluminum, which will help to increase the temperature.

It is essential to use food-grade quality materials for the screens or racks. Ideally one should use screens made of stainless steel, Teflon-coated fiberglass or plastic. Avoid screens made of copper, aluminum or "hardware cloth" which is basically galvanized metal coated with zinc or cadmium. All these metals are unsafe since they can oxidize, leave residue on food or affect the nutritional quality of food items.

To protect the drying fruits from birds and insects, it is important to protect the fruits with some form of covering. To do this, one can simply use either another screen or a covering of cheesecloth.

## Solar Drying

Solar drying is the result of technological advances made in the field of sun drying. Solar drying is a process of drying foods by harnessing the heat energy of the sun in a special dehydrator that not only increase the temperature but also, improves the air flow. This speeds up the process of drying the food and reduces the risk of food getting moldy or spoilt.

A solar dryer increases the temperature by using a reflector such as glass or aluminum while air flow is improved with the help of vents at each end. The technique and system is fairly simple. Cool air enters the dryer, removes moisture and escapes. The reflector surface helps to increase the heat by 20 °F to 30 °F. A cover of plastic protects the food, prevents rain or dew from dampening it and screens over the vents prevent birds and insects from attacking the fruit.

One may need to change the position of the solar dryer throughout the day in order to maximize the heat received from the sun. Also, one will have to stir the food several times to ensure uniform drying.

Solar dehydrators are available easily and in many variants. One can even make them at home after getting the requisite directions.

## Vine Drying

Vine drying is yet another simple and effective way of drying food outdoors. This method is especially useful for beans and lentils. All one needs to do in order to dry beans such as kidney, soy, lima, navy and lentils, is to leave the bean pods on the vine till the beans inside rattle. It is relatively simple since no pretreatment of food is required. Once the bean pods are completely dry, simply pick them and shell. If required, further drying may be completed by drying them in the sun, oven or a commercial dehydrator.

## Pasteurization

It is important to treat fruits and beans dried in the sun or on the vines and kill any insects and their eggs. One can use any one of these two methods for this purpose. The first is the freezer method. For this, one can simply seal the dried food in freezer plastic bags and place them in a freezer set at 0 °F or below and leave them at least 48 hours. The second is the oven method. For this place the food in a single layer on a tray or in a shallow pan, and then place the tray or pan in an oven preheated to 160 °F for 30 minutes.

## Drying Foods Indoors

Drying foods indoors is easy and possible with the help of modern gadgets such as food dehydrators, conventional ovens or countertop convection ovens. While one can dry herbs in a microwave, it isn't possible to dry other foods simply because there isn't adequate air flow.

## Food Dehydrators

Food dehydrators are small electrical appliances that can be used to dry and preserve food indoors. A dehydrator has an electric element for the heat and a fan and vents for air flow and circulation. Most dehydrators are designed to dry foods at 140 °F, which makes them efficient and quick.

These days, one can buy a food dehydrator from department stores, natural food stores, mail-order catalogs or garden supplies stores and catalogs. Dehydrators can cost anywhere from $50 to $350 or above depending on features. While most have standard features, some models may be expandable with provision for extra trays. The only possible disadvantage that a dehydrator may have is its limited capacity and therefore, expandable dehydrators may be a better option.

## Dehydrator Features

- Double wall construction of metal or high-grade plastic with enclosed heating elements and an enclosed thermostat with temperatures from 85 °F to 160 °F.

- A dial for regulating temperature and a timer to prevent food from over-drying and scorching.

- An easy-to-use, counter top design.

- A fan or blower to ensure flow of air and circulation.

- Four to ten open mesh trays made of sturdy lightweight plastic. Trays should be easily washable and low on maintenance.

- The UL seal of approval with a one-year guarantee.

- Easy to maintain and use with proven after-sales service.

## Types of Dehydrators

Usually, dehydrators come in two designs where one has a horizontal air flow since the heating element and fan are located on the side while the other model has a vertical air flow with the element and fan located at the base.

Dehydrators with a horizontal flow of air have several advantages – mixing of flavors is reduced which allows several foods to be dried simultaneously, there is no dripping of liquid or juices and all trays are heated equally. Vertical flow dehydrators cannot prevent mixing of flavors and this can increase the time for drying different types of foods.

## Homemade Dehydrators

 It is possible to build a dehydrator at home after getting the required instructions from the county Extension offices. A homemade dehydrator will be cheaper however; it may not be as convenient and efficient as a commercial one.

## Oven Drying

An oven can easily and effectively be used to dry food. Ovens have all the three elements needed for food drying – heat, low humidity and air flow. However, while it can be possible to dry small amounts of fruit leathers, meat jerky, banana chips or mushrooms, it is indeed difficult to use a home oven to dry large quantities on a regular basis.

Moreover, drying food in the oven is a slow and time-consuming process. Most ovens do not have an in-built fan and therefore, they end up taking more time and energy to dry relatively small quantities of food.

## Room Drying

Drying food in the room is different from sun drying. Here the food that has to be dried is placed in a well-ventilated room or covered space. Fruits, nuts, herbs and hot peppers are usually dried in this manner.

To dry herbs and hot peppers, either suspend them from a string or tie in bundles and suspend them from overhead racks. Keep the herbs and peppers covered in paper bags with small openings to allow air circulation. The paper covering will protect them from dust, insects and other pollutants. To air dry nuts in the room, simply spread them on a single layer of paper while for partially sun dried fruits, one can simply leave them on their drying trays.

## Dehydrofreezing

Dehydrofreezing is a new method of food preservation that uses both the techniques of drying and freezing. Fruits that have been dried at home usually have 80 percent of their moisture removed while vegetables have 90 percent. However, if only 70 percent of the moisture is removed and then, the fruit or vegetable is stored in the freezer, the final product will definitely be better tasting. Dehydrofreezing achieves this by combining freezing and drying.

However, it is important to understand that dehydrofreezing is not the same as freeze-drying. Freeze-drying is an expensive commercial technique that creates a vacuum while the food is freezing. This technique of food preservation cannot be performed at home.

In dehydrofreezing, the foods are partially dried and then, frozen. The low temperatures in the freezers prevent food from mold, bacteria and general spoiling. Moreover, since they have been dried, they take less space. In addition, the taste and color of such foods is definitely better than foods that have only been dried. Another great advantage of dehydrofrozen foods is that they reconstitute in about one-half the time it takes for dried foods, making the former a quicker and easier option.

## Packaging and Storing Dried Foods

It is important to pack and store dried foods properly since they are prone to insect contamination and moisture re-absorption.

Begin by cooling the foods completely. Foods that are warm tend to give off moisture, which could cause mold and bacteria. After cooling, tightly pack the dried food into clean and dry insect-proof containers. While packing them tightly, do ensure that the food does not get crushed or broken.

One can use glass jars, metal cans, boxes with tight fitted lids or moisture-vapor resistant freezer cartons to pack foods. While it is possible to use heavy-duty plastic bags, these cannot protect the food from insects and rodents. To keep out moisture, use plastic bags with a 3/8-inch seal. Fruit that has been sulfured should not be placed in metal containers directly. Fumes from sulfur can react with the metal and cause discoloration. So, place the fruit first in a plastic bag and then, store it in a metal canister.

It is a good idea to pack foods according to serving -or recipe-size amounts. Reopening the package several times will expose the dried food to air and moisture, therefore reducing its shelf life and quality.

Store dried food in cool, dark areas and most dried foods have a storage time from 4 months to a year. The storage temperature plays an important role in determining shelf life. Higher storage temperatures mean lower storage time. Most dried fruits can be stored for a year at a temperature of 60 °F and for 6 months at a temperature of 80 °F. Dried vegetables can be stored for half the storage period of that of fruits.

Keep a close eye on stored dried food to check for moisture that may creep in during storage. Glass containers make this easily possible. If one spots moisture on food, it is a good idea to dry and package them again. Moldy foods, however, should be discarded immediately.

# References

- Food-preservation, sports-and-everyday-life-food-and-drink-food-and-cooking: encyclopedia.com, Retrieved 23 July, 2019

- Preservatives: foodadditivesworld.com, Retrieved 16 June, 2019

- Preserving-Food-by-Drying: partselect.com, Retrieved 14 March, 2019

- Trigo M. J.; Sousa M. B.; Sapata M. M.; Ferreira A.; Curado T.; Andrada L.; Veloso M. G. (2009). "Radiation processing of minimally processed vegetables and aromatic plants". Radiation Physics and Chemistry. 78 (7–8): 659–663. doi:10.1016/j.radphyschem.2009.03.052

- Pearce, L.E.; Smythe, B.W.; Crawford, R.A.; Oakley, E.; Hathaway, S.C.; Shepherd, J.M. (2012). "Pasteurization of milk: The heat inactivation kinetics of milk-borne dairy pathogens under commercial-type conditions of turbulent flow". Journal of Dairy Science. 95 (1): 20–35. doi:10.3168/jds.2011-4556. ISSN 0022-0302. PMID 22192181

- McGee, Harold (2004). On Food and Cooking: The Science and Lore of the Kitchen. New York: Scribner, pp. 291–296. ISBN 0-684-80001-2

# Permissions

# Index

CPSIA information can be obtained
at www.ICGtesting.com
Printed in the USA
BVHW060920030622
638819BV00003B/15

9 781647 401504